Face Your Acne

10 Holistic Ways to Eliminate Acne

Estrellita Gonzalez

She Power Publishing

Canadian Cataloguing in Publication Data:

Gonzalez, Estrellita, 1964 -
Face Your Acne
Ten Holistic Ways to Eliminate Acne
ISBN-13: 978-1540509260

She Power Publishing
2786 West 16 Avenue, #206
Vancouver, BC
CANADA V6K 4M1

Release date: September 25, 2016
Typeset, printed and bound in Canada

DISCLAIMER

QUOTES

Be good to your skin. You'll wear it every day for the rest of your life ~ *Renée Rouleau*

I'm a big believer in that if you focus on good skincare, you really won't need a lot of makeup

~ *Demi Moore.*

Nature gives you the face you have at twenty; it is up to you to merit the face you have at fifty ~ *Coco Chanel*

DEDICATION

This book is dedicated to the many acne clients we have had the privilege of serving over the last several years at my holistic skin care clinic, Derma Bright Clinic. Your battle with acne inspired me to write this book, to provide the information and suggested treatment ideas to combat this often insidious condition.

To be a teenager is a glorious time in a person's life. It is a time of a growing awareness of the person you are becoming. It is also a challenging time, full of physical growth and changes that can be difficult and lonely.

My hope is that the words in this book will inspire teens to take control of their health, resulting in not just radiant, glowing skin, but an improved overall sense of wellbeing and health.

You have one body, treat it as a temple and it will provide you with a life of wonder, energy and longevity.

This book is also dedicated to my son, Enrique. I really wrote this with him in mind as he starts his journey into "teenagehood". I hope this book will give you advice and assurance that maybe sounds better coming from a book than from "mom". Love you Enrique!

Live long and prosper!

Love and light,

Estrellita Gonzalez

FOREWORD

In my 35+ years as a medical beauty therapist, I have observed many changes in the applications for skin and body care. These applications include the use of mecnanical, chemical and nutritional studies to change our appearances at some level. Despite all the new technologies to give rise in the quest for eternal youth, it comes at a price.... both monetary and, in many cases, physical pain.

Youth and health always start from the foundation that evolved from our ancestors and is established prior to conception. However, the care within the womb and the care after birth set the stage for the rest of one's life.

Every cell in our body responds to both the internal and external stimuli. Sometimes I like to refer to this as "internal and external hygiene". How, when and what you feed to the "internal and external hygiene" will always determine the outcome in your appearance and health.

When your foundation is strong and solid, you can recover naturally and quickly without much assistance. However, should your foundation be weak, you will need sufficient external assistance to repair it; many times the damage is so severe that nothing will help.

Our nutriments can either be our medicine or our poison. What is tolerable for others could be our poison... always listen and feel your body's reactions.

Before I make recommendations to my clients for home care, I like to see the natural state of the skin in order to get to the root cause of the problem. Often I assess their nutriments, sleep and cleansing routine during the consultation (which may include a service) and suggest changes over a two week period of time.

Observations within this two week period often are quite dramatic as the body has the natural ability to regenerate and heal when given the correct tools and environment. The effects are long lasting and should there be any post pigmentation indications then I will recommend other technological treatments such as LED or laser.

For best results your professional therapist should have a decent understanding of the physiology of the body, chemical and physical applications and medical devices. Your body will respond accordingly to:

- What you eat;
- How you think, and
- Who and what your surroundings are.

Hence, always listen and be good to your body as it will always talk back.

Sandra Mah
Senior Medical Beauty Therapist
CIDESCO DIPLOMAT 1989

PREFACE

I operate a holistic skincare clinic in Vancouver, BC, Canada. I have operated this business for almost five years now. I am not an aesthetician, I run the business focusing on the marketing and operations side. From the day I started this business I wanted to create a centre devoted to healing from the inside out coupled with the use of new, non invasive natural technologies.

I feel strongly that our skin is a reflection of what is going on inside our bodies. Whether it be a mature person dealing with the signs of aging or a young person dealing with acne, the usual culprit is inflammation, and a result of the choices we make in relation to diet, lifestyle, stress and others factors.

I especially want to help teenagers who are feeling terrible about themselves due to their acne. We live in a society obsessed with glamour, beauty and youth. When you don't fit in because you have acne, it takes its toll on a young person and their self esteem. I had acne as a teen and I remember how awful it felt to feel different, and flawed. In our teens this is compounded by our already fragile self-image.

I decided to write this book for parents who have kids dealing with acne. Although anyone can read it and take its points into practice, it is often the parents who embark on the healing journey for their children dealing with acne.

As the parent of a teenage son myself, I felt compelled to share my knowledge and tips so that parents can arm themselves with information to implement the small changes that will inevitably result in clearer skin for their teen, as well as a happier teen overall.

Please enjoy the book and I welcome your comments, please free to connect with me!

Estrellita Gonzalez
Owner, Derma Bright Clinic
www.dermabrightclinic.com

INTRODUCTION

Why is good skin so important? Why do we spend so much time and energy striving for clear, bright, youthful, healthy skin and are willing to do almost anything to get it? I believe there are two reasons. First, our face creates a first impression, and fortunately or not, we are often judged by it. Secondly, our skin is a reflection of what is going on inside our bodies. I feel that at a biological and genetic level, we gauge our fellow tribe members' health by the state of their skin. Our skin reflects how we are feeling and is a barometer of our health so subconsciously we know that skin reflects our state of health and wellbeing.

I own and operate a holistic skincare and slimming clinic, Derma Bright Clinic, in Vancouver, BC, Canada. One of our specialties is acne. It is often heartbreaking to see our young clients come in with a face full of acne. Our mission is to help these clients achieve healthy bright skin. This book was written to give parents of teens helpful information to achieve this goal. With knowledge, coaching and the right services and products your teen will achieve this goal!

I have divided this book into two main areas: first, an overview of acne including its symptoms and triggers, and second, a list of healthy habits your teen can adopt today to start bringing out their best and brightest skin!

By educating and then following the tips, I believe you and your entire family will be well on your way to achieving the skin you want!

WHAT IS ACNE?

Okay, so your teen has acne, but what is it really?

According to the Canadian Dermatology Association, acne occurs "when hair follicles become clogged by a combination of an oily substance (produced by the skin) called sebum, dirt, and dead skin cells. Often, bacteria called Propionibacterium acnes (P. acnes) can be present which can contribute to the redness, swelling and pus that can accompany lesions. The visible result is acne, which is the term used to describe blackheads, whiteheads, pimples, and cysts. Acne usually appears on the face and neck but it can also develop on the shoulders, back, and arms."

Generally, healthy pores shed one layer of dead skin cells per day inside the pore, but acne-prone pores shed up to five layers of dead skin cells per day (hyperproliferation); I have even heard heard up to a billion cells per day in some individuals! In this case, the body cannot keep up with keeping the pore clean, the cells become sticky and get stuck inside the pores and forms a plug. Also, the P. acnes bacteria is fed by the sebum and proliferates (though it is not the cause of acne). The ultimate cause is too many dead skin cells.

A little know fact is that acne takes 30-90 days to form. A pimple you see today started as a microcomedone (see below) 3 months ago. It will take 3-4 months to see your skin clear up and it means 3 months worth of acne is going to surface. What your teen needs to do is to start a regimen that is going to keep the new acne from forming so s/he will not see it surface 3 months from now. Skin also needs time to adapt and the regimen will need to change as the skin changes. A skincare professional can help with this process so it is advisable to get an assessment so your teen can see where s/he is at.

It is important to note that 85% of us in the western world will experience acne!

Types of Acne

There are two main types of acne: teen and adult.

Teen acne: Starts as a result of a surge in sex hormones that happens at puberty. Male hormones (androgens) increase the size and number of sebaceous glands as well as the amount of sebum (oily substance) they produce.

Adult acne (acne tarda): Defined as acne that develops (late-onset acne) or continues (persistent acne) after the age of 25. It is more common in women.

Acne Causes

Acne is generally caused by too many dead cells in the pores, overactive sebaceous glands that produce more sebum (oil) which then clogs pores and can lead to inflammation (redness and swelling).

Genes can be another factor - if either parents had acne as a teen your teen will most likely also develop it. But not all people will experience inflammation as this is an inherited tendency.

Everyone can get a pimple somewhere on their body sometime in their lifetime. Acne often starts around puberty and may last 5-10 years or it can continue into adulthood. Even some babies develop acne shortly after birth (due to hormones from the mother).

Acne Breakdown

The following are some of the terms associated with acne:

- **Comedones (plural for comedo):** are plugged follicles.There are two types:
- **Open comedo:** a blackhead as the surface is visible and turns "black" when it's exposed to air. Blackheads can become infected or not depending on whether the P. acnes bacteria have affected the cells around the pore.
- **Closed comedo:** a whitehead, which is like a blackhead, but is closed at the surface.

- **Plugged follicles & Bacteria:** follicles can become irritated and swollen enough to burst, thus affecting surrounding tissues. The plugged follicle can erupt above the skin's surface. The sebaceous material (oil) in the pore contains a lot of P. acnes bacteria and this infects the surrounding area when it erupts, creating a red bump known as a pimple.

- **Pustule:** different from a pimple as it contains white blood cells which work to fight off the P. acnes infection; these pile up and create pus in the pore.

- **Nodule:** a deeper inflamed solid dome-shaped lesion that forms below the surface, deep into the skin's layers.

- **Cyst:** when a group of pustules cluster together under the skin they form a cyst, and these are pus-filled and can have a diameter of up to 5mm. They are usually very painful and scarring is common.

There are basically four levels of acne severity:

- **Mild acne:** a few lesions that are close to the surface, and not deep or inflamed;

- **Moderate acne:** marked by deeper nodular lesions and some redness;

- **Severe acne:** many lesions, multiple cysts, a great deal of redness & inflammation, and

- **Cystic acne:** lots of pustules, nodules, papules and cysts along with severe breakouts and inflammation.

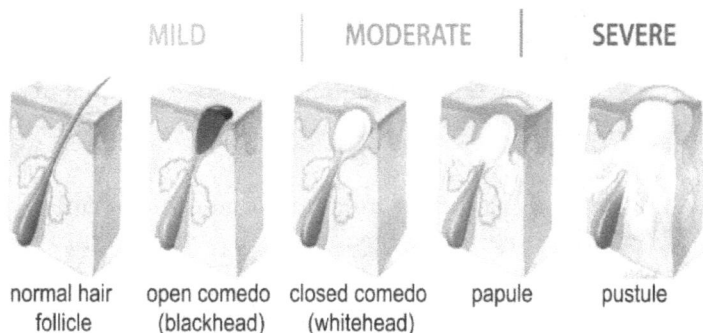

MILD | MODERATE | SEVERE

| normal hair follicle | open comedo (blackhead) | closed comedo (whitehead) | papule | pustule |

Cystic Acne (Photo © A.D.A.M)

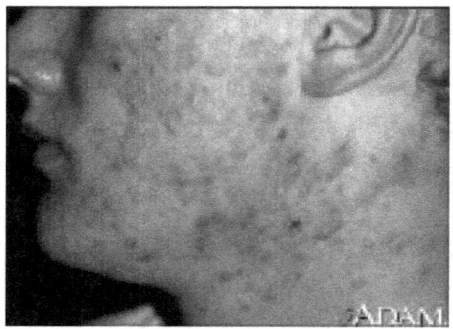

Common Symptoms

For teen acne, common symptoms include:

- Acne on those regions of the body with the most oil glands including the face, neck, chest, back, shoulders and upper arms.

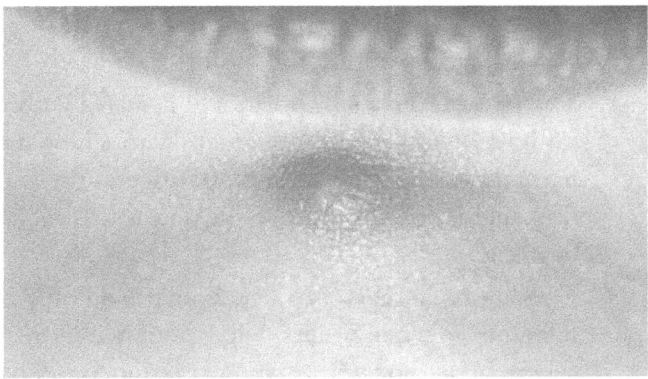

- Lesions will include clogged pores (pimples, blackheads or whiteheads), papules, pustules and/or cysts.

- The most easily treated and least severe are blackheads and whiteheads.
- With severe acne, a grade 4 for instance, often medication would be required to treat inflammation, bacterial infection, redness or pus.
- For adult acne, common symptoms include:

- Inflammatory acne in the lower facial region or macro-comedones (microcysts) spread over the face.
- Hormonal breakouts/spots on the chin and/or jaw line that mainly become more inflamed during the premenstrual stage of a woman's cycle (the week before her period).
- An oily T-zone area (centre of the brows, nose and chin) with dry and flaky cheeks.
- A pattern where the breakouts tend to be more dominant on one side of the chin one month and likely to be more noticeable on the opposite side

next month with a period of improvement for about 2 weeks during the month.

- The pattern relates to hormonal changes within the body, as the hormones fluctuate with a woman's natural cycle it affects the oil balance in the skin, thus increasing the feeding ground for the acne bacteria.

- Conditions do vary as some women will only notice a few spots while others will experience more severe breakouts with cystic breakouts (under-the-skin lumps usually seen on the jaw line).

PH Balance

Skin has a barrier called the acid mantle and problems arise when this is damaged through picking, over strenuous or abrasive cleansing and using harsh products. The acid mantle houses the sweat and sebum and generally needs a PH of 4-5. A lot of soaps contain harsh detergents that can destroy the delicate balance of the PH either increasing or decreasing it thereby making skin weaker and more susceptible to infection.

Causes

Again lots of ideas on what the actual cause of acne is but I believe it is related to three main areas that can work together (or in extreme situations, separately):

- Hormones;
- Toxic Buildup, and
- Hereditary factors

Hormones

We know that teenagehood is associated with hormone changes. Puberty brings on the increased production of Androgens which stimulates more oil production in the skin. Add in the possibility of improperly eliminated used hormones which work to over stimulate the oil glands as well and it will result in having oily skin. The passive acne bacteria P. Vulgaris can be activated if fed blood toxins which then compounds the situation. To help counter this hormone onslaught one can help the body fight these hormones by producing more Prostaglandins, which are biochemicals that communicate with hormones. They will help androgen hormones stay in balance by regulating hormones. More on this later!

Toxic Buildup

We live in a toxic world. From the air we breathe to the water we drink to the food we eat, all of these are not as pure as we would like. Many of our bodily processes leave some toxic remnants which must be eliminated on a daily basis. There are things we need to do every day in order to eliminate this toxic buildup; these will be addressed in a later chapter.

Hereditary

There is a genetic link for acne. So chances are that if the parents had acne, then the teen will most likely as well. The good news is that parents today did not have the level of information that we now have in relation to acne and how to treat it!

Other Acne Triggers

There are a variety of factors that can trigger acne flare ups and/or lead to breakouts. Consider avoiding these things if you notice that they make your teen's acne worse:

Cosmetics: Hair and makeup products can clog pores. When purchasing products look for acne-friendly terms on labels such as non-comedogenic, non-acnegenic and oil-free.

Physical pressure: Pressure due to a chin strap, phone receiver, sports helmet, headband, guitar strap, bra strap and other tight clothing can lead to localized acne that develops at the point of skin contact.

Sweating: Can worsen acne as it helps to clog pores, especially if trapped under clothing.

Over-washing: Washing the face twice a day with a mild cleanser is recommended for acne-prone skin. Cleaning it more often, scrubbing/exfoliating, or using strong cleansers or astringent products (i.e. toners with alcohol) can actually strip the skin and irritate it, which can lead to more acne.

Menstrual cycle: Many girls and women may notice that their acne flares up as they are nearing their monthly period.

Food: There is some conclusive evidence that certain foods aggravate acne; if your teen experiences a reaction try removing it from their diet for a period of time. Sugar feeds bacteria so it should be kept to a minimum.

Touching the skin: We do this several times a day if we do not pay attention, often with dirty hands. Each time we do this we transfer germs to our skin. Also when we touch our hair and then our face, we transfer hair fats and impurities. Pay attention to this.

Medications: Certain medications can cause flare ups such as oral corticosteroids, contraceptive pills and anti-convulsions.

Using cosmetics not suitable for the skin type: We are inundated daily with beauty products that promise all sorts of miracles. We do not need most of these. If you do decide to purchase something be sure the ingredients are well-suited to your teen's skin type and condition.

Using a mobile phone: In a study in 2009 that involved 200 hospital staff, researchers found that 94.5% of the phones were contaminated with some kind of bacteria. A lot of the bacteria had been transferred by the user's hands to the phone. Gross! Most of us use our phones for 2+ hours a day so it is critical to keep it clean. Use a natural disinfectant to wipe the phone clean a few times a day and use earphones as much as possible.

Hot Showers and baths: The hot water here can remove the sebum layer from the skin's surface thus dehydrating your skin. Use "warm" water instead and use a light moisturizing cream after getting out of the shower.

Sleeping on the stomach: This puts pressure on the skin as it is pushed against the pillow; it can also cause premature wrinkles.

Dirty makeup brushes: Each time your teen uses a makeup brush they leave makeup, sebum and dust on the brush. Keep them clean by using a natural cleanser or shampoo to wash them weekly.

Using expired products: All beauty products will have an expiration date so do not use them if expired as they may lead to developing more sensitive skin.

Smoking: This is a no brainer really but we will point out that smoking can decrease capillary and arteriolar blood flow which could damage connective tissues that are important for healthy skin. Smoking also damages the skin's fibroblasts which are important in the formation of collagen and elastin; as a result, smokers will experience premature aging and are at a higher risk for psoriasis.

Holistic Approach

There is always new research coming out on ways to treat acne. The rest of this book highlights ten major areas to help your teen clear their acne holistically. This list is suggests practices that we recommend daily to our clients when treating acne.

Truly the best solution to eradicate acne is a holistic one. Acne is a reflection of an imbalance in the body and by treating it holistically, that is by treating the whole body, your teen will set himself up for success as well as help their entire body be its best, in how it operates as well as how it looks and feels.

We live in an ever changing world and the way how we are treating illnesses and afflictions offers people a number of choices. I believe in the need for both allopathic or conventional medicine as well as in natural medicine; I believe the two can coexist. There are major differences in the two approaches, however.

Conventional medicine looks at the body as separate parts and thus tends to treat it separately. It does not always look to cure its patients, but rather help them to live with the condition comfortably. It also relies heavily on pharmaceuticals which in my opinion tend to only deal with the symptoms and not get to the root cause of the illness. Many of these drugs are also synthetic, something our bodies just do not care for or know how to process. Often there are side effects from drugs which can require additional drugs to treat those symptoms, a vicious cycle if you ask me.

Natural medicine looks at the body as a whole, and looks to balance it and create an environment that supports the body healing itself. Examples of natural medicine include Naturopathy, Homeopathy, Ayurveda and Traditional Chinese Medicine. I like these philosophies better as I would prefer to be rid of a condition entirely than simply manage it using drugs. This is the issue I have with acne treatments. Many Dermatologists simply recommend drugs and even Accutane (yikes - see my opinion on this later in the book). This is not the answer. A more holistic way exists and through the next several chapters I will provide ideas on how to do just that!

SKIN CARE STRATEGIES & ROUTINE

I t is critical to establish a consistent skin care routine. Acne starts with microcomedones so your teen needs to prevent them from forming in the first place. A proper professional consultation and home care routine can help with this.

Professional advice

If you are starting to notice your teen's skin changing, especially in relation to acne (see previous symptoms), it is vital that you seek professional help as quickly as possible.

Dermatologists are usually the first choice to go see, though they are getting more and more difficult to get into see (where I live in Vancouver, it can be up to a year before you can get an appointment). The Dermatologist pattern is common: oral antibiotics, topical antibiotics, and/or prescription retinoids. Sometimes benzoyl peroxide is recommended or if this fails, a cycle of isotretinoin. Often none of these will work. Research has shown that patients do not follow the regimens and that more frequent visits are associated with increased compliance; this is where an Aesthetician can make the difference.

A professionally trained Aesthetician can spend more time with your teen and be the coach and cheerleader through this more holistic process, and without the use of medication. Initially a treatment protocol would include visits every two weeks for a two to three month time frame. It is important though that you do your research here. Not all Aestheticians are equal. Training varies and many do not know enough about skin and skin issues. Before you go see one, review their web site and credentials so that you are comfortable in going to them with your teen's skin issues.

- As an example, our typical treatment program involves the following steps:
- An initial assessment to meet, discuss and learn about your teen's lifestyle, use of medications, drugs, makeup, food and skin care products;
- Review of a strict home care and treatment plan as well as follow up to ensure what is expected of your teen;
- A plan designed around the type and severity of your teen's acne;
- Ongoing coaching and assessment of your teen's skin during subsequent sessions;

- Extractions with each office visit to help clear your teen's skin quickly;

Blue LED Light treatment, and

- Possible exfoliation or peel treatment.

Dermatologists are necessary if your teen suffers with severe acne; Aestheticians cannot treat class 4/severe acne but they can treat classes 1, 2 and 3.

Professional services

An Aesthetician should always start with a complimentary Skin Assessment followed by suggested treatment protocols. The following are some recommended services including:

- **Acne Exfoliation and Extractions**: Exfoliation is a very important part of treating acne as it removes dirt and dead cells and allows for the penetration of products. Extractions will be necessary in the beginning of the treatment course but will become less necessary as the program progresses.
- **Corrective peels:** For acne scars (not severe) and dark spots (hyperpigmentation). Peels aid in sloughing off dead cells; using Alpha hydroxy Acids (AHA's) in the form of fruit acids made from milk, cane sugar, apples, and oranges will dissolve dead cells making skin more luminous and smooth. We like to use herbal peels as well for this.
- **Blue LED Light**: We use Blue LED light in our treatments as it has been proven to kill the P. acnes bacteria often present on acneic skin. Treatments are

pleasant, pain-free with no down time. Blue light is also a proven mood enhancer!

- **Oxygen**: Another tool we like to use is the application of a stream of pure oxygen as it kills bacteria and aids in healing the skin re any inflammation and redness.

Home care routine

When putting together your teen's home care routine, an Aesthetician would be looking for the following:

- Look for the right acne product for your teen's type of acne. A product for inflamed acne i.e. pimples, pustules, etc would not be suitable for non-inflamed acne e.g. blackheads.
- The products need to be strong enough for your teen's skin type. If they are not, your teen's skin will not change much; if too strong it will irritate or dehydrate the skin, and cause breakouts.
- Use the products in the right way: you need strong products to get the acne under control, but if your teen uses too much too soon it will irritate or dehydrate the skin. Start slowly.
- Account for skin adaptation. This means to not let your teen's skin get too used to the products or it will stop responding and not get clear.

Skincare products

The following is a suggested list of skincare products to use as part of a home care routine:

- **Cleanser**: Use a high-quality, gentle face wash rather than a creamy cleanser. Use lukewarm water and let the cleanser sit on the skin for a few seconds to break down any dirt and makeup. The cleanser should be sulphate and paraben free and perhaps have a small amount of salicylic acid to help exfoliate and decongest the skin. Cleanse twice a day, once in the morning and once before bed.

- **Toner:** If your teen is using a good wash s/he will not need a toner. Acne skin needs to stay cool; a toner can help with this. It is also important to work on maintaining the moisture that is in the skin and to keep inflammation down. Use once a day in the mornings.

- **Moisturizer:** Use a light, more liquid moisturizer. This is where a lot of people go wrong, choosing something that is too heavy for acne-prone skin. A suitable moisturizer should be quick to absorb and water-based (or "oil-free"). Even for someone with dry areas, such as cheeks, this will help. It may take a week or two to see an improvement. Use a small amount, spread it as best as they can and be patient. Your teen could also add a serum for acne to this as well. Use once or twice a day as needed.

- **Sunscreen:** Once this routine is down, add a high quality chemical-free sunscreen (at least 30 SPF) or mineral powder. More on this later!

- **Exfoliation:** Look for a "clean" facial Exfoliant and use it twice a week, in the mornings. There are several things your teen can use: scrub (ideally a gentle agent such as jojoba beads), a brush (natural bristle brush), an exfoliating cleanser such as a physical exfoliator (with organic scrubbing beads or a chemical exfoliator (with salicylic or glycolic acids). We are fans of natural products; avoid anything synthetic i.e. some exfoliators have plastic beads, which are bad for the skin as well as the environment. Exfoliate twice a week.

- **Makeup remover:** I am a big fan of coconut oil and it easily wipes off eye makeup and mascara. Coconut

oil has antimicrobial and antibacterial properties and is safe for the eyes.

For those with more active acne issues, look for two choices of active ingredients that can be added to a moisturizer: salicylic acid and/or glycolic acid. Care is needed when using these ingredients, instructions must be followed and ideally consult a skin care professional to recommend what would best suit your teen rather than buy products over the counter.

If these ingredients are over-used or the strength is too much for the skin it may result in increased dryness. Most skin care clinics offer a free consultation so take advantage of this. Ensure your teen is being advised what products are best for the skin type, age, condition, etc and then you have someone to call if your teen experiences any problems with the products.

Essential oils

I am a big fan always of natural and organic ingredients. I also believe that essential oils can be a great help in dealing with acne and other skin issues. Here are some suggestions:

- **Oregano oil:** just a drop on a breakout can speed up healing and prevent scars.
- **Lavender oil:** Is the perfect aid to a number of skin issues. It is great for treating inflammation, burns, sunburn, wounds, scars, wrinkles, insect and animal bites as well as skin issues such as acne, eczema, psoriasis and more. Here are some suggested recipes courtesy of Julia Thomas of http://vivohummingbird.com/

- **Sunburn**: Mix a few drops with apple cider vinegar and distilled water in a cobalt blue spray bottle and spray on affected areas frequently. Also, a cool bath with a few drops added along with some apple cider vinegar.
  - **Burns:** Apply a few drops of lavender to the burn and cover up immediately. Do not put cold water on a burn as it will blister!
  - **Sunscreen:** Make your own! Add lavender, carrot seed and geranium essential oils to melted beeswax, coconut oil, olive oil and sesame oil with a little zinc oxide.
  - **Sleep:** Lavender is a fantastic sleep aid! Add a few drops to your pillow, or place on the back of your neck or tips of ears!
  - **Tea Tree oil:** Is an immune stimulant and antiseptic. It fights bacterial infection, viral and fungal infections. It only targets harmful bacteria and leaves beneficial bacteria alone. Great for spot treating acne.

FOOD

I cannot stress enough the importance that food plays in the acne riddle. There is enough evidence available now to support that diet and acne are related. Much of this centres on how what we eat affects the hormones which will thus trigger acne symptoms such as increased oil production, hyperproliferation and inflammation.

This is probably the most difficult area for an acne sufferer to contend with. The reasons are many, from not knowing food triggers, to having to give up comfort foods and make those hard, healthier choices. But, if your teen truly want better skin, s/he has to face their acne head on and the battle with their favourite foods.

My suggestion is to designate a certain period of time such as 2 - 3 months to eliminate some of the trigger foods outlined here so your teen can make room to try some of the others outlined in this chapter. Keeping a food journal will also be really helpful to monitor the triggers as well as document the symptoms and eventual clearing of many of these symptoms.

Insulin-like Growth Factor (IGF-1)

Teenagers are notorious for not eating well. Their diets tend to be laden with high (bad) fat, sugar and carbohydrate rich foods. The problem is that a lot of these foods result in an increase in Insulin-like Growth Factor or IGF-1. This substance is now believed to promote acne in a similar way as insulin by creating Hyperkeratosis, a thickening of the outer epidermis which blocks the excessive sebum from flowing to the skin's surface. This can later lead to the formation of a cyst. Studies conducted on post-adolescent women aged 20-25 with acne found increased levels of IGF-1. The bottom line, what teens are eating does chemically affect acne.

Foods to avoid

So let's get the hard stuff out of the way right off the bat!

There have been extensive studies conducted on two primary acne-promoting dietary factors: dairy and high glycemic load foods. These foods influence inflammation and hormones which increase acne prevalence and severity. Any hormonal influences that raise insulin and/or insulin-like growth factor 1 (IGF-1) are important here as these elevations can lead to gene expression changes linked to inflammation, oil production, acne lesion development, and more. These changes have also been linked to certain cancers such as breast and prostate. You can see why maintaining and balancing hormones becomes important!

Here is a list of what to avoid, at least for a period of time (2-3 months ideally):

Dairy: Numerous studies have found a link between milk consumption and acne. One study cited involved nine, 15 year old girls who experienced a 20% increase in acne prevalence; these girls consumed two or more servings of milk per day compared to fewer than one per week. It was the same for all types of milk from whole to skim. Similar results were found in a study of boys who drank skim milk. Dairy causes mucus to form and coats the digestive tract which slows the absorption of nutrients. It can also lead to sinus and yeast infections; remember that yeast feeds off sugar. Casein, which is one of two proteins found in dairy, has also been linked to cancer. Dr. T Colin Campbell, author of the China Study, found through his studies that casein is the most relevant cancer promoter ever discovered and has links to a number of health issues ranging from respiratory and digestive issues to acne.

High-glycemic load foods: Ok, a little science here, sorry! As a definition, Glycemic Load (GL) is a measure of the effect of a certain food on blood glucose levels. High-GL foods such as refined carbohydrates produce dangerous spikes in blood glucose, leading to excessive insulin levels in the blood which contribute to heart disease, diabetes, and cancer. These spikes not only promote inflammation but also raises IGF-1 levels, which contributes to acne. A low glycemic load diet has been shown to improve acne symptoms, and decrease IGF-1 and skin oil production in several studies. The two most important hormonal factors that drive acne are IGF-1 and insulin. Have your teen avoid high-glycemic load foods, especially sweeteners and commercial baked goods, and make sure they get an adequate supply of micronutrients through whole foods including fruits and vegetables. Remember, high glycemic carbohydrates can raise both insulin and IGF-1.

Oil: Excessive oil production by the skin can be exacerbated by oil intake. Vegetable oils drive omega-6 intake up, which have pro-inflammatory effects, and high omega-6 intake is associated with the development of acne. The effects of oil intake on acne is exacerbated by the consumption of high glycemic carbohydrates, such as commercial baked goods. So do what you can to avoid oils such as canola, peanut, safflower, and the like. Aim to use olive oil for dressings but not to cook with as it turns bad with high heat. Use coconut oil for high heat cooking.

Wheat: Gluten affects a lot of people, and not in a good way. There are glutinous proteins found in wheat, barley and rye (called Prolamins) that can make your gut permeable, meaning some of these proteins can get into your bloodstream affecting your immune system and causing inflammation. Both of these will aggravate acne. It will also allow other gut bacterial parts and proteins (casein) to do the same. It is best to avoid gluten and other lectin-containing foods such as potatoes, corn and rice, altogether. Wheat has shown to damage the small intestine (leading to nutritional deficiencies), increase the toxic body load and gluten specifically to cause inflammation. Avoid things like bread, cakes, pastas, basically anything made of wheat!

Sugar and Refined Carbohydrates: Diets high in these are the worst causes of acne. This has to do with the insulin surges mentioned previously. They also increase inflammation in the body and upset the bacterial balance in the gut. Acne sufferers put on low glycemic diets have shown significant improvement both in acne and insulin sensitivity.

"High androgen" foods: These include things like peanuts, peanut oil, peanut butter, corn oil, wheat germ, shellfish, organ meats (e.g. liver, sweetbreads, heart) as these contain hormones that can make acne worse.

Iodides/salt: This category includes foods, vitamin supplements and sports drinks/bars. Food examples include iodized salt, seafood, fish, seaweed, fast foods, and dairy products (cows like to lick iodized salt licks). Iodides and chlorine are common pool disinfectants which can remain in the water and cause skin issues for frequent swimmers. This coupled with hot and humid weather, physical exercise and pools all can cause acne flare-ups. Re dairy, milk and cheese contain Iodides as well as hormones that contribute to acne. Health foods and supplements may contain some form of iodides and/or biotin in the form of iodine, iodide, potassium iodide or kelp. Protein bars often have potassium iodides and watch protein powders such as whey and soy - use hemp or pea protein instead. Vegetables to minimize include asparagus and broccoli; they should not be eaten every day as they are high in iodides.

If you are seriously interested in helping eliminate your teen's acne, you need to eliminate sugar, grains, cereals, potatoes, corn, rice, pasta, and processed foods from their diet.Fruit, because it is high in fructose (a natural sugar) should be minimized. Berries are low in sugar so they are fine. Avoid all fruit juices unless you are juicing yourself and including the whole fruit or vegetable (for its fibre).

And please note that chocolate and greasy foods do not aggravate acne. Chocolate, specifically dark, is an anti-oxidant and so has health benefits! Just watch the sugar intake!

Balanced diet

An imbalance occurs in the body when it is not being fed proper nutrition. Nutritional deficiency is how most disease occurs as the body does not receive enough building blocks and energy to balance itself.

Unfortunately the Western diet is not a clean, wholesome diet. Look around any mall and see the number of fast food outlets all touting their over-processed, unnatural food. These foods are full of refined and simple carbohydrates, dairy, hydrogenated fats and acid-forming components. All of this dysfunction wreaks havoc with our digestive systems resulting in poor evacuation of waste through the overloaded waste organs, and ends up coming out through the skin, especially if dealing with hormone issues as well.

Several studies have been done on various indigenous populations around the world who consume fruits, vegetables, nuts, fish and other whole foods and acne is just not present in these cultures. What does this tell you? In North America we are not eating the right foods for our health.

What should we be eating?

A balanced diet is a combination of high quality complex carbohydrates, "clean" protein sources (no farmed fish, eat grass fed meat whenever you can), fibre, healthy fats, lots of vegetables, and some fruit. See the Nutritarian chart in the Appendix for a clear example.

Foods to eat

There are plenty of foods your teen can eat that will help acne and provide many other benefits as well. The following outline suggestions for the minerals, vitamins, and fats to consume along with food suggestions.

Minerals, fats and vitamins:

Omega-3 fatty acids: Prostaglandin 3 or Omega 3's are associated with reduced likelihood of acne, as omega-3s counteract the pro-inflammatory processes that drive acne. So it will calm irritated skin providing a smoother complexion. Omega-3 fats will help to normalize skin lipids and prevent dehydration in the cells. This will keep skin cells strong and moisturized. Great sources include salmon, fish oils (check your labels and purchase the higher quality versions), chia and flax seeds, and walnuts.

GLA (Gamma-Linolenic Acid): Found in borage and evening primrose oils. GLA is very effective in producing Prostaglandin E1 which is the powerful anti-inflammatory hormone that helps with immunity and fighting inflammation as well as inhibits the production of pro-inflammatory hormone Prostaglandin E2 which aggravates acne. Take this along with antioxidants, zinc, Vitamin B complex and lecithin to help the GLA convert. Please note that dairy and wheat have been found to inhibit the production of Prostaglandin E1 and promote the creation of Prostaglandin E2.

Good fats: Just because overeating nuts and oil (especially peanuts and peanut butter) can contribute to sebum production and acne, does not mean that all nuts and seeds need to be eliminated from the diet. It is the combination of the glycemic load of the diet with other hormonal promoters acting together that produces acne. So excessive intake of fat may increase sebum production, but this tendency is permitted and exacerbated by the glycemic effect of the diet. If your teen's diet is free of high glycemic carbohydrates, it can tolerate more fat, without any acne-promoting effects on sebum production, because the antioxidant and phytochemical exposure is higher, and the glycemic load of the diet is lower. Good sources include avocados, walnuts, cold water fish and coconut oil.

Fibre: Eat greens, whole grains, chia seeds and oats.

Vitamins: A, B, C, E for cell regeneration. Many acne sufferers are often low in vitamins A and E especially. Vitamin E is a fat soluble vitamin and protects Vitamin A and EFA's from oxidation. Add sunflower seeds, dark leafy greens, olive oil, nuts, avocados, fish, broccoli and kiwis.

Sea Buckthorn: I have heard interesting things about this ancient herb. A wild form of it is said to have 190 bioactive substances including vitamin E and the richest source of carotenoids on the planet! One of the Sea Buckthorn oil's qualities is its ability to lower testosterone overproduction common to males. It is also an anti-inflammatory and one of the best EFA's for the acne prone.

Vitamin D: Important for maintaining a healthy immune response. Most people are deficient in it, especially the more north you go. Without adequate vitamin D, your body cannot fight infection, in your skin or elsewhere. Exposing large areas of your skin to appropriate amounts of sunshine is the best way to optimize your vitamin D levels. If you cannot do this supplement with Vitamin D3 drops. I take 3,000-5,000 IU's! Foods include krill and herring.

Zinc: Studies have shown that acne sufferers are low in zinc. It is a proven anti-oxidant as well a killer of bacteria, inflammation and reduces the keratinocyte activation.

Some general food suggestions:

Hemp and flax: These are high in zinc and so are beneficial.

Fruits: Blueberries, strawberries and papaya: these are a great source of enzymes and antioxidants.

Protein rich leafy green vegetables: a great source of vegetable protein and antioxidants.

Green smoothies: Use dark leafy greens as the chlorophyll is good for us. Your teen can rebuild their skin with green smoothies.

All vegetables: With a special emphasis on beans, greens, onions and mushrooms.

Raw nuts and seeds: Up to two ounces can generally be eaten by those on an oil-free diet without creating acne. But once one starts eating refined and high glycemic carbohydrates, the body will be more sensitive to the fat in the diet, maybe even from nuts.

Protective micronutrients: Tests have shown that the blood levels of zinc, carotenoids, and vitamin E are lower in acne sufferers when compared to those without acne. This suggests that a diet rich in micronutrients may help prevent acne. Carotenoids can be found in green and orange vegetables, and vitamin E is found in nuts and seeds. Pumpkin seeds and hemp seeds are rich in zinc, but zinc absorption efficiency may be low on a plant-based diet so it is advisable to take a mineral and/or multivitamin supplement to assure optimal levels of zinc, iodine, vitamins D and B12.

Salmon: Its high omega-3 content helps hydrate skin from the inside out and reduce the inflammation that can cause skin redness.

Antioxidant-rich foods and drinks: Such as blueberries, blackberries, dark greens, green tea and coffee, help fight free radicals that can damage the cellular structures of the skin.

Tomatoes: Are rich in Lycopene, another antioxidant that can combat free radicals (molecules or ions that can damage healthy cells and suppress the immune system); tomatoes help protect against some cancers, including lung cancer.

Kale: This popular leafy green is a major source of vitamin K (one cup cooked contains almost 12 times the recommended daily value), which may help ward off heart disease and osteoporosis.

Eggplant: The deep-purple skin gets its rich color from nasunin, a nutrient that helps fight the spread of cancerous cells by cutting off the blood supply they need to multiply.

Red Bell Pepper: This immunity-boosting superstar contains roughly 60 percent more vitamin C—which triggers the production of white blood cells that fight off germs and bacteria—than its green counterpart.

Basil: One of the herb's medicinal properties comes from the antioxidant eugenol. Recent lab studies found that this compound sparks anticarcinogenic activity in cervical cancer cells, causing them to self-destruct.

Brussels Sprouts: Our cells are naturally equipped with tumor-suppressing genes, and the sulfur compounds found in brussels sprouts may help those genes by blocking enzymes that promote tumor growth. A 2012 study also found that these sulfur compounds could play a key role in treating rheumatoid arthritis by reducing inflammation and activating cartilage-protecting proteins.

Nutritarian diet

Hundreds of people with severe acne, of all ages have resolved their acne, and gained a healthy colorful glow to their skin by following a Nutritarian diet. This diet, coined and developed by Dr. Joel Fuhrman, MD is defined as a diet that is nutrient dense, rich in plants and includes cancer fighting superfoods. The richness in antioxidants protects against acne and gives skin a healthy color and more youthful appearance as one ages. See the Appendix for handouts on this diet.

A word about fruit and juice. Fruit has natural sugar as well as vitamins, antioxidants and fibre. Juice is just sugar, so better to skip it all together. Fibre is often overlooked but very important for a lot of body functions especially in relation to our digestion. It also helps us to feel full and is beneficial for lowering heart disease. Aim for an intake of 25 (women) to 38 (men) grams a day.

Becoming a bit of a "foodie" will serve one well in life. Sound nutrition really is the basis of a healthy, vibrant body which of course will help skin immensely. Get your teen interested in the food s/he is eating and look for healthy, wholesome recipes that will be good for their skin and body. Green smoothies are a great way to start the day especially when your teen is first working on clearing their acne. Start with a morning smoothie for a week and see what changes.

The best approach to food is eating a balanced diet that includes the foods your teen's body needs including healthy carbs and fats. A third of our daily calories should come from high performance fats such as Omega-3 fats in fish, nuts and vegetables. Low fat foods are not good for us and often contain loads of sugar so they taste "good".

Food testing

It may be worthwhile to explore food sensitivity or allergy testing for your teen. A food allergy is the result of the body's reaction to a food it thinks is an invader. Our body works to deal with it by sending in the immune systems which then results in allergic symptoms. This adds more stress of course to our already taxed liver.

Testing can help to identify the foods your teen may want to avoid. It can be done through either a Naturopath, Allergist or Holistic Nutritionist; it is often surprising to see the results. I did this early in my own health journey and was surprised to find certain foods such as soy and peanuts on the list, especially as I rarely ate soy!

Cleansing and fasting

If your teen has severe acne, it may also be worth exploring a fast though I would encourage you to do this under the guidance of a professional such as a Naturopath, Nutritionist or Traditional Chinese Medicine Practitioner. I like to do a bit of a cleanse at least once a year and there are lots of ways to do this. You can visit a natural food store for assistance or try a company which offers different options.

It is an idea to remove certain trigger foods such as wheat and dairy for a period of time. Try for a week or ideally up to at least four weeks (this is when a food diary is also very helpful). Other common trigger foods include soy, gluten, sugar, nightshades and processed foods. Many people do experience issues with these foods including bloating, breakouts, inflammation, rashes and low energy. Pay attention to the difference in your teen's skin when you take time to cook meals at home, eating more vegetables, whole grains, raw nuts, and fresh fruit? Does his skin change? How is her energy? Mental acuity? Emotions? Once you remove these trigger foods from their system, reintroduce them, one at a time. Your teen may notice an allergic reaction such as itchy eyes, stuffy nose, or sneezing which may occur within the first 90 seconds of eating. Also watch their mood and see if you notice any change.

It is a good idea to limit stimulants such as sugar, coffee and alcohol. And watch to see if your teen may have a bit of a reliance or addiction to these. Look at their relationship to these stimulants and help them make changes if you realize there is something not balanced here. These can also wreak havoc on their kidneys and liver as well as joints, and energy levels. Try to stay within a moderate level and do a detox if you think there is an issue. Sugar is one of the most common and is certainly worth considering to reduce in their diet; their taste buds will change!

Eating raw

There are times when our bodies need to detox. The start of an acne breakout may be a great time to try several detoxifying methods including juicing, fasts, and eating raw. I am not espousing this as a lifestyle but it is something to try when your teen needs to re-balance his or her body.

Eating raw can have many skin benefits. Our skin is our largest organ and it is an important barometer as to our overall health and well-being. One of the keys to bright, clear skin is a diet rich in fresh, organic (if possible) fruits and vegetables. When you eat raw food your body receives more essential vitamins, amino acids and water naturally. Cooking eliminates a large amount of water from vegetables.

When your teen starts eating raw you will notice changes such as feeling generally better, having more energy, and they will look better. People will start to notice and your teen will look and feel their best naturally all around.

Supplements and testing

Earlier I mentioned some important supplements to take including Omega 3's. It may be worth consulting a Holistic Nutritionist or Naturopath to get some systemic testing done to see if your teen is low in any important vitamins such as A, B, C, D and others. Vitamin D is so important for general health. Did you know that the further north you go the higher the cancer rates per capita? What is the connection here? Less sun of course! So those of us in the north need to supplement with Vitamin D to make up the shortfall we are not able to get from the sun. Recommended Daily Allowances (RDAs) are 400 IU's which is very low. During the winter I will take 4,000 to 5,000 IU's.

I often suggest people over 40 get three tests: Heavy Metals, Food Sensitivity and Hormone. Though these are not probably as relevant for acne, they can serve as a wonderful blueprint for your teen's health.

IV injections can be very worthwhile for anyone who is chronically deficient and these can be administered by a Naturopath. Our internal organs, especially the liver, are often abused with an overload of toxins from hormone therapy (eg birth control pills, HRT), topical products, household cleaners and an array of other chemicals found in everyday things such as cleaning products. Take care of your liver! I start my day with a glass of water with some fresh lemon, a great way to detox the liver on a daily basis!

We had a client we were treating for acne and he was doing great on our system. A few months later he came in and his face had exploded with acne. Our Chief Aesthetician immediately saw that something was off and suggested to the mom to take her son to a Naturopath to get tested. Sure enough, he had Leaky Gut Syndrome! His body was not getting the nutrition it needed so it went into damage control mode. Once they found this out he was able to get on a treatment protocol that eventually led to a drastic reduction in his acne again.

"We are what we eat" is one thing but we have to make sure what we are eating has the proper nutrition too. This is why eating organic has its place as it has been found that organic food has denser nutrition than non-organic. I realize that eating organic can be expensive so I suggest purchasing organic foods that are high in toxic pesticides and herbicides. And generally anything you can peel is safer than something without a peel. In other words go organic for non-peeled fruit such as strawberries and red peppers, but go non-organic with bananas and oranges! The EWG publishes its list of "the Dirty Dozen", foods to avoid purchasing; the list this year includes strawberries, celery, tomatoes and grapes! The the "15 clean list" includes pineapple, avocados, kiwi and eggplant.

GMO foods

I feel the need to talk a little about Genetically Modified Organisms foods (GMO). What is GMO? It is "the result of a laboratory process of taking genes from one species and inserting them into another in an attempt to obtain a desired trait or characteristic, hence they are also known as transgenic organisms".

It is "frankenfood"; food that has been modified in a laboratory usually for herbicide tolerance or the ability of a plant to produce its own pest resistance. Many of the processed foods in the North American diet are made of GMO foods and most people have no idea.

Why is this bad? We do not know the full effect of these foods on our bodies as they have never been tested. The only feeding study done with humans showed that GMO's survived within the stomach of people eating GMO food; no follow up studies were done! Lots of animal test have showed pre-cancerous cell growth, smaller brains and other ghastly effects.

There are a number of side effects ranging from plants creating toxins to the creation of new proteins inside the plant. The bottom line is that the effects of consuming these new combination of proteins are unknown. And we know there has been a surge in autoimmune disorders, gastrointestinal diseases and more. I firmly believe that GMO foods are at the root of this problem.

Common GMO foods include:

- Three main US commodity crops including field corn (92%), soybeans (94%) and cotton (94%);
- US sugar beet is over 95% genetically modified for herbicide resistance;
- In Canada, 98% of canola is genetically modified for herbicide resistance, and
- Other common crops include papaya, zucchini, squash, alfalfa, and some potatoes and apples.

There is a long list of "invisible ingredients" as well, ranging from baking powder to whey powder. For a list go here: http://nongmoshoppingguide.com/brands/invisible-gm-ingredients.html

It is critical that you look for "non-GMO" on the label of your food product purchases and if you are not sure, ask the retailer!

STRESS

Stress is not good for anyone and for the acne-prone teen it stimulates the adrenal gland and releases cortisol which promotes oil production and then clogs pores. It also weakens the immune system and depletes vital minerals and vitamins in the body including magnesium, potassium, vitamins B and C.

Stress also affects the liver, weakening it and affecting its ability to regulate the hormones which are already causing problems for the acne sufferer. Stress can also kill the good bacteria in the gut and make blood more acidic.

High levels of cortisol are also known to inhibit the production of collagen as it overrides the enzyme collagenase which determines how much collagen is released to a traumatized area of the skin which can lead to insulin resistance in the epidermis.

Psychological stress can also lead to oxidative stress and inflammation which means more pimples.

Given all of this I highly recommend your teen take proactive actions in managing his stress.

De-stressing techniques

- The following are a variety of techniques to manage stress:
- **Breathe work:** oxygen is nourishing and relaxing;
- **Meditation:** a relaxed mind benefits in so many ways;
- **Massage:** one of the best things to do for the body is a regular massage practice; it is awesome for detoxing and moving lymphatic fluid;
- **Talk it out:** talk to your teen about having them confide in friends or family when they are stressed out;
- **Exercise:** raising the heart rate once a day makes skin glow. Exercise improves circulation and oxygen capacity, and it will improve the complexion. Skin also has endorphin receptors, which help one feel positive afterwards;
- **Small luxuries:** treat oneself when having had a success in your day;
- **Mindset:** this is a big part of a wellbeing practice; look for ways to keep self talk positive, and use visualizations and affirmations to create a great life;

- **Self Care:** take time to take care of yourself, without guilt;make yourself a priority and be okay with that!
- **Delegation:** when you can, delegate!
- **Coach:** for life, business, success; even a coach needs a coach!
- **Addiction management:** look at your teen and identify whether s/he may have issues with addictions such as smoking, marijuana and alcohol consumption; if so, help them seek help;
- **Detoxing:** we live in a toxic world so we have to be proactive in detoxifying on a regular basis. Some ideas include lymphatic drainage, using a rebounder, infrared sauna, exercise, massage; all of these will aid in detoxing the body from food, allergens, pollution, hormone therapies such as the birth control pill, etc. Perhaps look at a liver cleanse; our organs share biochemical pathways and a happy liver reflects in healthy skin;
- **Yoga:** an excellent stress reliever as it promotes stretching, breathing and relaxation. Everyone can benefit from synchronizing the breath with movement, exploring balance and focus, setting an intention and finding flow. This could be the start to working on a mind-body practice that will serve your teen well in life.
- **Emotional Freedom Technique or EFT:** this involves tapping the body's energy meridians with one's fingertips to clear emotional blocks which then restores a balance to the mind, body and spirit.
- I call stress the silent killer. Everyone has stress in their lives but the secret is how to manage it. Deal with stress, and your skin will not be the only thing that

improves! Your teen will have better relationships, better sleep and her sense of overall well-being will be greatly improved.

Mindset

If your teen is serious about clearing her acne she needs to adopt a tough mindset as it may not be an easy process for her given some of the changes to diet she will need to make. Help her be resolute in her desire to change and have her commit to the process 100%. The toughest part to any kind of desire to change is the mental toughness it will require.

Some ideas to do this:

- **Identify first what it is your teen wants to change:** have him ask himself "what am I not happy about?" It may be very helpful to start a journal about this question. Have him spend some time daily to ponder his situation. "What am I unhappy about? What do I stress about? What makes me feel sad, frustrated, anxious, or unhappy?" These are perfectly normal emotions. Remind him that he is in control of them but he has to acknowledge them first. Everything starts with awareness!

- **Make a list of goals:** Once he has done some self exploration, have him start to make a list of the goals he would like to achieve. Use the SMART process; I have outlined a goal using this format: Goal: I want to clear my acne 80% by the end of 6 months:
  - Specific: make the goals as specific as possible;
  - Measurable: use numbers as I did above:

- Attainable: is the goal achievable? Unrealistic goals are hard to get excited about!
- Relevant: is the goal relevant to your teen and the situation? Does he really want to achieve this goal?
- Timely: establish a timeline as most people are motivated by a deadline.

- **Educate oneself:** Now that your teen has a clear set of goals for the situation, he can start to educate himself to fill in the missing information. If he is wanting to achieve the goal above, he now has the resources he needs (through this book!) to get out there and educate himself!
- **Take action:** And with education established your teen can now go ahead and start taking action! She is in control, no one else so encourage her to go ahead and do what she needs to do! She will be happy with herself as she checks in and sees the progress she is making as she follows the plan!

SLEEP

Sleep is vitally important to overall general well-being. For the acne sufferer, a lack of sleep increases hormone levels which may result in breakouts. Your body detoxifies itself while you sleep; the liver works to eliminate toxins from the blood which otherwise may be reabsorbed into the body and emerge through the skin, not what you want!

I recommend that clients aim for at least 7 - 8 hours a night; teenagers will need more e.g. 10-12 as their bodies are growing. The body does its healing while asleep so getting adequate sleep is absolutely necessary for optimal health and wellbeing.

Sleep deprivation is very harmful to the body. Studies show it can shrink the brain, cause one to eat more and increase blood pressure. Cortisol, the stress hormone, ages the skin and can cause acne. Sleep reduces the cortisol level in the body. So it's a simple equation: Sleep = younger, clearer skin!

Sleep is not optional! It is necessary to get the adequate number of hours!

To ensure your teen is getting the right amount of sleep it is helpful to start by creating the right environment and atmosphere in their bedroom.

<u>Helpful hints</u>

There are a number of things your teen can do to create that perfect sleep environment:

- Create a sleep ritual!
- Remove distractions such as electronic devices from the bedroom;
- If your teen uses electronic devices at night, leave at least an hour of no use before going to sleep;
- If your teen must keep their cell phone nearby, have it at least 10 feet away from their head to avoid exposure to electrosmog and turn the ringer off;
- Do not keep a TV or computer in the bedroom;
- Have them change their sheets regularly; this is critical for pillows as they will attract and hold the oil from skin and hair and this will aggravate skin;
- Keep their room tidy as clutter makes it difficult to sleep;
- Keep their room dark, the darker the better, and
- Have them avoid caffeine at least 3 hours before bed.

Helping them create an oasis in their bedroom will allow for a better sleep and your teen will feel so much better when they awake refreshed!

Here is an awesome interview about sleep with two of my favourite online ladies: Arianna Huffington & Marie Forleo. This interview is about Arianna's book on sleep, the Sleep Revolution! So much has been learned about sleep in recent years and Arianna is bringing this to the forefront!

Check it out here:http://www.marieforleo.com/2016/07/arianna-huffington-sleep-revolution/

Here are some highlights for me of this interview:

- One of Arianna's points that is worth repeating is that our brain is very frenetic at night while we sleep. For years we were told our brains were still at night and now we understand it is the opposite! What is it doing? It is cleaning up the toxins in our body that accumulated during the day! Wow! Who knew?!
- We need 7 - 9 hours of sleep on average.
- Value sleep, make it a priority and commit to yourself to do so daily.
- Have a ritual and transition period like we did when we were kids. Remember those days? Bath, pajamas and a story, then off to bed. We lost that somewhere along the way as adults so create your own.
- Remove all electronic distractions from the bedroom. If you have a TV in your bedroom just commit to not watching it before bed.
- Right before you go to sleep, think of the things in your life that you are grateful for. I do this every night and I feel it is a great way to go to sleep,

thinking positive thoughts which should translate to happy dreams!

- Have a sleep kit with you at home and for when you travel. It can include things such as an eye mask, noise cancelling headphones, lavender spray, soothing teas, and sleep meditations and programs on your ipod.

Great suggestions and as I always say, everything starts with awareness so now go forward and help your teen make those changes!

TOXIC OVERLOAD

What are toxins

As mentioned previously, toxins are everywhere, many of which can't always be controlled. What we have some level of control over though is the toxic load affecting our bodies and environment.

In Bruce Lipton's wonderful book "Spontaneous Evolution", he discusses the "new-edge science" of epigenetics which centres on the notion that an organism's biology and genetic activity are influenced by its interaction with its environment. He posits that rather than being victims of our genes by controlling our environment we have the power to "control our biology and become masters of our fate." What I take from this is that we have a lot of control over our health by looking for ways of managing our environment and its potentially toxic residue.

It is important to point out that a relatively small percentage of disease can be attributed to our genetic predispositions. The US National Cancer Institute has determined that at least 60% of cancers originate from environmental causes.

For us humans, a toxic buildup can happen when the body's organs of elimination, namely the liver, kidneys and intestines, cannot handle the large amounts of waste produced. This then affects the blood, bowels and puts a heavy burden on the liver. Let's be clear, most people have overloaded livers and completely neglect its care. But acne sufferers have the added burden of all the hormone issues going on. When the organs cannot properly eliminate as they are taxed, the lungs and skin become the mechanism to do so.

Overloaded bowels result in a mucus buildup which can feed parasites and candida. When the liver is not functioning at its optimal, toxins derived from cell waste, bad food, etc are not expelled properly and are reabsorbed into the blood.

What is detoxing

Detoxing can be as simple as cleaning up the diet. The idea with a detox is to take a period of time to eliminate certain foods and perhaps add a cleanse, juice or fast program. I would only encourage this action with the guidance of a trained alternative medicine professional such as a Naturopath, Traditional Chinese Medicine (TCM) Doctor or a Holistic Nutritionist.

A word about using alternative types of healing modalities. We are fortunate in Canada to have access to a decent allopathic medical system. And we are fortunate to have have access to complementary medicine options as well. In the US, half the population visits complementary physicians as alternative healing methods have proven to be effective, less expensive and a lot safer than allopathic medicine. The Chinese and Ayurvedic traditions have been around over 4,000 years for a reason! These practices see the body as a quantum holistic system and work to restore the body's natural balance and harmony. When this is achieved, the body's terrain discourages dis-ease or disease-producing disturbances.

Although there are many opinions about these types of alternative procedures, to me it is common sense to give our bodies a rest once in awhile from the work of processing and digesting foods. Perhaps even a break from meat once in awhile can offer a lot benefits to the body. Alternative practitioners in my opinion are just better informed in how to manage these types of activities for optimal results.

Detoxing Organs

There are several of the body's organs involved in detoxing. These include:

- Liver: During a cleanse, the liver needs to rest. It is the most important detoxifier as it neutralizes and filters toxins from other parts of the body as well as its own.
- Colon: The primary waste eliminator. Even during a fast or cleanse the colon will dispel waste including acids and toxins.
- Kidneys: An important eliminator of fluids and purifier of blood. Drinks lots of clean water during a cleanse in order to flush the kidneys well.
- Lungs: Every breath you take is absorbed and expelled by the lungs and contains toxins. Deep and yoga type breathing helps with toxin elimination.

- Skin: the body's largest organ. It takes a lot of abuse, so during a cleanse, help it by brushing, cleaning and scrubbing it. Avoid synthetic clothing, take hot/cold showers and epsom baths to help intensify toxin elimination.

What to eat or not eat during a detox

If your teen is interested in trying a bit of a detox the following are suggested foods to eat and eliminate during a detoxing period of time:

- Eat: Broccoli, sprouts, blueberries, onions/garlic, carrots, watermelons, apples, spinach, grapes, avocados and nuts/seeds.
- Protein: Many vegetables contain protein. Nut milks and wheatgrass are also great sources of protein during a cleanse.
- Bacteria replacement: During a cleanse it is important to replace the gut flora. Check with your practitioner but good sources are acidophilus, bifidus and yoghurt.
- Liquids:
- Apple cider vinegar: Raw and unfiltered apple cider is a terrific antiseptic drink and is a powerful cleanser that works to maintain the right acid/alkaline balanced in the intestines. I like to take 2 tablespoons in the mornings in water or use it on salads.
- Herb teas: There are many therapeutic and nutritional herb teas such as peppermint, chamomile, and rose hips that can provide hydration and relief of symptoms such as nausea.

- Greens: Wheatgrass and other green vegetables are great healing agents due to chlorophyll and antioxidant components.

- Water: A powerful flushing agent and cleanser. Make sure to drink pure water; avoid, tap, distilled and spring waters, Add lemon juice as it stimulates the digestive area.

Digestive enzymes: Help by encouraging the breakup of plaque and encourage absorption of nutrients.

Do not eat: Any kind of meat, dairy, fish; all refined carbs, white sugar, processed foods, caffeine, wheat, chocolate, alcohol, tobacco, fried or cooked meals, grapefruit (it affects the production of liver detox enzymes).

What to expect

There is a good chance that your teen will experience some discomfort during a cleanse program. This is a natural part of the elimination process, when the body works to regenerate and then expel waste through the elimination channels. Depending on the cleanse your teen decides to do, it may result in the dying of bacteria and parasites, a process which can lead to the release of ammonia and toxins. This is bound to result in your teen not feeling very well, but again it is a normal result of the cleanse process.

Common detoxing symptoms include headaches, fever, breaking out in whiteheads, diarrhea, irritability, mental depression, nausea and weakness.

It is important to remind your teen that things will get worse before they get better!

How long the process will last will depend on several factors, from the severity of the acne to the condition of your teen's elimination organs. It helps if your teen can set aside the time to do this, perhaps over a period of time such as a week, as there is a process the body will go through.

There are three stages to detoxing:

- Cleaning/rebuilding of vital internal organs: can make your teen tired and weak.
- Catabolism stage: the body works to release waste material, chemical and hormone residues, etc into the blood and lymph systems. Here your teen may experience a worse acne breakout.
- Anabolism: the body works to build new tissues. This may result in increased energy levels.

For best results, your teen is advised to rest plenty and to accept that the feelings and symptoms are a normal part of healing. The process may take up to 16 weeks for the full detox symptoms to abate.

Activities

During a cleanse or fast there are a few activities to include to help with the process:

Exercise

I mentioned exercise earlier but I will bring it up again here as it is critical for overall wellbeing. High-intensity exercise helps flush out toxins in the body and through the skin's pores. It provides oxygen to the skin's cells through increased blood flow, therefore, promoting healing. It balances hormone levels and also releases feel-good hormones. And the internal organs benefit with assistance in the expelling of toxins. We can all benefit from this!

During a cleanse or fast, be sure to reduce extreme physical activity and aim to do more gentle forms such as yoga, swimming and walking.

Infrared Sauna

When I found out I had lead poisoning one of the first things I did was purchase an infrared sauna! I love my sauna. It helps me detox, it burns 300-600 calories in a 20-30 minute session and leaves me feeling warm and peaceful. And it is great on a cold night! Most gyms today have one so encourage your teen to try one out. S/he will feel great and lessen their toxic load!

Fragrance

A word about fragrance. Most are synthetic and many contain hundreds of ingredients which are not listed on labels. Often there are harmful chemicals that are just not good for us. Fragrance is the cause of many issues from asthma and rashes to allergies and migraines. Try to mitigate as much as possible the use of fragrance.

Suggestions include using fragrance-free laundry detergents, and avoiding the use of fabric softeners and sheets, especially on pillow cases as they cause a waxy residue that can clog pores. Limit the use of air fragrances for home or car and also on the skin; instead use pure essential oils.

Cleaning products are another area to watch for. Remember, clean does not have a smell! Despite the marketing campaigns, cleaning products do not smell like lemons or lavender.

DIGESTIVE HEALTH

Accoording to Biomic Sciences, a well known supplement manufacturer, 70% of the immune system is located in the gut. This is something most of us are not aware of. What we do know is that the immune system is the key and foundation to better, overall health and wellbeing. Thankfully consumers are starting to be proactive around their health rather than reactive and this will benefit all of us as we work towards a healthier society.

When it comes to our digestive health there are many things we can do starting with eating more natural and functional foods. I consult with a variety of practitioners around things people can do to help with their skin. One is Holistic Nutritionist, Sharon Pendlington of www.personalnutrition.ca who sees acne in some of her clients as well.

The following are some thoughts and ideas from Sharon and others in relation to acne and its connection to gut health.

As we know, skin is an organ of elimination as well as protection. When other elimination organs such as the liver, kidneys and colon are overloaded, excess toxins are secreted through the skin resulting in acne and other skin issues.

When people go to the doctor for their acne, conventional medical treatments can include a variety of things including Accutane, which in my opinion is poison (see that last chapter on my thoughts). Many of these options will often leave the skin peeling and drying (from prescribed topicals), with gut dysbiosis which is overgrowth of poor gut bacteria (from antibiotics) as well as nausea, headaches, vomiting and depression from oral medications.

I have mentioned in previous chapters the influence of toxic accumulation as well as hormone fluctuations on acne; other causes include stress, excess iodine, high arachidonic acid levels (from high meat protein), low levels of zinc, Vitamin A, Vitamin B6 and Essential Fatty Acids.

Holistic Nutritionists can help acne sufferers in a couple of key ways. Firstly they can assess the digestive, intestinal, kidney, lymphatic and endocrine systems to help get to the root cause of the inflammation. The assessment (which can be as easy as a hair analysis) can reveal overloaded organs or dysbiosis. With this information a diet or lifestyle modification plan can be developed to reduce the toxic load and help with symptoms. For hormone imbalances, there are food changes that can help with overloaded adrenal glands.

A hair analysis can also help identify mineral deficiencies related to iodine and zinc as these can also cause skin lesions; this can be remedied with supplements.

Some helpful Nutritionist tips for acne sufferers include:

- Eat a whole foods diet rich in whole grains, legumes, fruits and vegetables;
- Optimize digestion;
- Avoid the usual suspects including sugar, processed foods and animal fats;
- Eat the right kinds of proteins including eggs, fish, and plant-based protein;
- Deal with chronic stress, and
- Alkalize the diet with leafy, dark green vegetables.

How optimizing your gut can help acne

So we know that the gut plays an important role in general health and wellbeing. It also plays a large role in acne.

When acne sufferers can make the dietary changes recommended the gut will naturally improve as well. There are things that your teen can take to help the gut as well including fermented foods which will encourage beneficial microorganism growth. What is interesting here is that these microorganisms communicate throughout the body including skin and gut mucosa. To reestablish bacterial balance incorporate fermented, cultured and raw foods (they contain living beneficial bacteria) into your teen's diet. A high-quality probiotic supplement is also an option and especially important if your teen has been on antibiotics. These drugs will indiscriminately kill off all bacteria, including the beneficial, resulting in a compromised immune system.

Stress and emotional health are also connected to the gut. Research by dermatologists John Stokes and Donald Pillsbury posited that emotions can alter the microflora in the intestines which then affects inflammation leading to acne and other skin issues.

Hormones

I have addressed hormones in previous chapters. In addition to this, if possible, women should aim to avoid low-estrogen birth control pills, Norplant, Provera and Depo-Provera, as well as progesterone hormone replacement Premarin. Polycystic ovaries will cause hormonal changes and breakouts. Taking birth control pills may delay the onset of acne but once off them your teen may experience the acne she would have had before taking them.

Candida

Our aim here is to build a candida-free environment. What is candida? It is a microorganism and yeast that likes to hang out inside the digestive tract; it can turn into a fungus given the right environment. An overgrowth from candida produces a waste product called mycotoxins which can have adverse effect on immune systems, tissues, brain and especially the liver.

Common symptoms of a candida overgrowth are many including but not limited to:

- Recurrent urinary tract and or vaginal infections;
- Anxiety, depression, feeling forgetful;
- Heart palpitations, headaches and backaches,

- Indigestion, bloating, gas, belching, constipation and diarrhea, and
- Dry skin, rashes, psoriasis and eczema.

Candida likes an acidic environment; this means blood Ph is more acid than alkaline. We feel better generally when we are in an alkaline state (this means a more vegetable, fruit and whole food diet).

If you suspect your teen has a candida issue, deal with it immediately. Again, the best is to visit a Naturopath and/or TCM doctor. If your teen has candida and fixes this problem, you will see a noticeable difference in the acne, it may even disappear!

Candida Test

If your teen is interested to see if s/he has candida, try this test at home:

- First thing in the morning, on an empty stomach, fill up a clear glass with mineral or reverse osmosis water.
- Spend several seconds building up an amount of saliva and spit into the glass.
- Leave the glass aside for an hour.
- Mild candida: you will see strings of saliva that look like legs form down in the water.
- Advanced candida: the saliva will sink to the bottom of the glass.
- The goal is to have saliva float in the glass!

The gut is an area all of us needs to pay attention to. It serves as the foundation of health for everyone and for the acne prone it can be the starting point to curing acne.

COSMETIC & BEAUTY PRODUCTS

As the "Queen of Living Clean", I am a big proponent of choosing skin care, body and cosmetic products that are as "clean" as possible. What do I mean by "clean"? Just as there is now a movement to "clean" food, the same care and attention needs to be given to the products you put on your skin, body and hair.

Some of the key things to look for in products include preservatives (i.e. parabens, BHT, and BHA), mineral oils, synthetic fragrances, colours, and fillers. All of these things lead to toxicity and a build-up in the body of toxins can lead to a host of health issues including inflammation, erosion, skin issues and aging.

There are "hot lists" created by governments to highlight ingredients not to be used in the manufacture of cosmetic, skin and hair products. In Europe, anything that has been linked in any way to cancer is not allowed to be used. So the list compiled by the European Union has about 2,000 ingredients listed; in Canada the list has 500 and in the USA, there are 11. That's right, 11! What a difference. And in Canada we import a lot of US products so it is really important for us to know this.

Here is a list of Canada's Hotlist of "bad" Ingredients.

You and your teens have the power to vote with your dollars – look at ingredients and purchase products that are chemical-free, toxin-free and where it makes sense, organic. And support companies who are making products with integrity and a social consciousness.

Toxicity aside, it is also critical to not use cosmetics or hair products that contain pore-clogging ingredients to avoid. As an example, Retin A has the pore-clogging ingredient isopropyl myristate as its first ingredient.

Quality ingredients

When purchasing a "clean" organic product, ensure you are purchasing a certified organic product formulation. There are a number of new and exciting base ingredients available today for skin and beauty product ingredients. One of my favourites is coconut oil. Organic cold pressed oils such as coconut and almost are great moisturizers and they are solvent free and contain no GMO ingredients or pesticides! Synthetic oils such as mineral and petroleum can clog pores and cause breakouts; they are also potentially xenoestrogenic (more on this later).

I use coconut oil as my eye makeup remover daily. Everything slides off easily including my mascara! Try it, you will LOVE it! Coconut is also full of essential fatty acids (EFA's) so it works as an anti-fungal, antibacterial and antimicrobial lauric acid resulting in clean, nourished eyelashes!

So many products out there use harsh chemicals and fill up landfills e.g. disposable wipes. There is just no need for this anymore! Nature has some of the best ingredients right there for the taking, so why purchase expensive products that are full of terrible ingredients while polluting the earth?

Helpful hints:

- Look for 100% organic food grade skin care for the health of your skin;
- Look for a product that is a "certified organic product formulation" versus "made with certified organic ingredients"; the difference can be substantial. You want a product that is fully compliant, not partially. Look for level certification and not an ingredient.
- Some products that appear "natural" are often so processed they ultimately end up synthetic.
- Semi-natural ingredients can have potential health concerns. Extensive processing can lead to issues of safety and purity.
- We have no access to know how a product is processed. Processing ingredients with synthetic chemicals is strictly prohibited in a certified organic product so you have the guarantee of a purely organic formulation.

It is really important to realize that the use of synthetics long term, causes low level irritation which triggers an inflammatory response from the body. Chronic inflammation ultimately leads to free radical generation, cell damage, wrinkles and sagging skin. Not where you want to be in the future!

This of course has a direct impact on the acne teen as well. We now know that inflammation is an acne trigger so mitigate the toxic load and you will minimize the inflammatory response.

A very useful resource is the Environmental Working Group and its web site www.ewg.org. This organization is lobbying the US government in relation to a number of toxic elements in our society, from GMO and BPA to toxic ingredients in beauty products. As part of this web site there is the Skin Deep Database where they have reviewed and rated thousands of skin, beauty and sun products on a scale of 1 - 10. Take some of your current beauty products and see how they stack up on this invaluable resource!

Pinkwashing

I get really angry when I think of the companies that are out there producing toxic products even more so when they turn around and promote things like fundraising cancer campaigns. This is called "pinkwashing" and many of our large beauty companies are responsible for this despicable practice. Vote with your dollars people!

Read your labels

Anything you put on your skin goes directly into your body so remember this whenever you or your teen are applying a sunscreen, fragrance or cosmetic. You want to know what is in it first so read your labels and start learning what to avoid and what is ok.

I am so passionate about this subject that I created an online store where we offer clean skin, beauty and personal care products as well as supplements and health information; it is called www.myskinsalon.com. I have also branded myself as the Queen of Living Clean with the intention to educate others through workshops, writing and speaking about the importance of paying attention to ingredients.

As a society we have a vested interest in promoting health. We need to encourage our citizens to make changes, open our eyes, not trust that our governments are always doing the right things and be conscious of the manufacturers we are supporting. Change is possible, and it all starts with awareness!

SUN EXPOSURE

S un exposure is a sensitive topic these days. I don't pretend to be an expert in any way but I do have my own thoughts on sun and sun exposure.

I believe we need sun for general good health. Ideally if we took in 20 minutes a day, without sunscreen, and ideally before 10 am or after 4 pm, we would naturally allow our body to build up its immune system and protect against things like cancer. The main source of Vitamin D is sunshine and if we don't get enough we become vitamin D deficient which can lead to health issues including weaker bones, a compromised immune system and cancer. An interesting fact is that the more north you go, the higher the cancer rates are per capita. What is apparent here? Well less sun of course! So northerners especially need more vitamin D and ideally from the sun. If that is difficult due to seasons and weather then supplement with vitamin D; I take daily D3 drops usually 4,000 IU's. This is far above the RDA of 400 IU's but I feel my body does better with a maxed out vitamin D load!

When you are taking in the sun naturally, you want to limit it to 20 minutes as more than this would require some kind of protection, and there are a multitude of things available to do that now. From mineral powder and coconut oil to a variety of clean suncare products; there are "clean" choices now!

As the face is always exposed it does need extra care and attention. Direct sun on the face (beyond 20 minutes) will dry and damage the skin, exacerbate hyperpigmentation and cause premature aging. Warm climates with heat and humidity can make acne worse.

For many, a tan denotes health but you do need to be careful here not to overdo it as it will cause wrinkles and age spots. You would be better to find a natural, "clean" self tanner. Long term exposure to the sun can cause a number of issues from lesions and tumours to pigment issues and Elastosis which is an accumulation of excess elastin in the dermis layer of the skin. So to protect the face from prolonged sun exposure I do recommend a "clean" sunscreen. And when you are out in the sun best to avoid the peak times from noon to 4 pm. For the acne teen, they need a non-pore plugging option.

The sun explained

The sun releases two major rays, UVA and UVB. To remember the difference, think of this: UVA promotes aging and UVB promotes burning.

There are two types of sun protection: sunscreens, which rely on chemicals to absorb harmful UVB rays, and sunblock, which forms a physical barrier to prevent rays from penetrating the skin.

Sunblocks works against UVA as they usually contain either zinc oxide or titanium dioxide (more on this later). When purchasing your sun care products you want "broad spectrum" coverage as it will protect against both UVA and UVB rays.

Sunscreen

If sun is a sensitive topic then sunscreen is even more so! And with good reason. With the work of such organizations as the Environmental Working Group and others, we are learning more about the dark side of the industry. Every year the EWG releases its analysis of over 700 sunscreen products. It is shocking to see the results year after year. On average only 25% of the products evaluated passed the test for safety and efficacy. Over 80% offered inadequate protection against the sun's harmful rays or had toxic ingredients (see below for more on this).

As mentioned, there is a movement underway to pay attention to ingredients in our products. As you know this is a subject I am passionate about, so much so that I have branded myself as *The Queen of Living Clean* to help people understand the importance of reading labels and paying attention to what they are putting on and in their bodies!

A great resource again to check your or your teen's personal care products (including skincare and suncare) are clean is the Skin Deep Database. Here over 65,000 products have been reviewed and scored on a scale from 0-10 for toxicity. See how your products rate so you can make the right choice for your teen's skin health!

Some natural alternatives include:

- Vitamin E: protects the skin against UVB radiation, decreases the development of cancer, and helps to reverse signs of skin photo-aging;
- Vitamin C: apply it topically as it has proven protection against sunburn, limits sun-induced DNA damage, and speeds healing of sunburned skin. Helpful in delaying the onset of skin tumours and well as in reducing wrinkling from UVB rays;
- Green tea polyphenol epigallocatechin-3-gallate: protects against oxidative cellular and genotoxic damage from UVA radiation;
- Coconut oil: as the polynesians have been doing for centuries, using coconut oil to protect their skin from the sun's harmful rays.

There are two key ingredients that are used in many cosmetic and suncare products to block intense sun rays without seeping deep into the skin and to the bloodstream; these are titanium dioxide and zinc oxide. There are two forms of titanium dioxide, anatase and rutile. The anatase form releases harmful free radicals into the body when exposed to light. This exposure disrupts the DNA structure causing the skin to be more susceptible to outside threats. Indoor light can also trigger this release! The rutile crystalline form is opaque and often used as a colorant. Many companies do not label the type of titanium dioxide they are using so I would just stay away from any kind of titanium dioxide and use only something with the zinc oxide.

Zinc oxide is a mineral that actually sits on top of the skin and works to scatter and reflect UVA and UVB rays. In my opinion it is much safer and effective than other ingredients.

Also make sure you are not using any form of nanoparticles as these enter the body and bloodstream, and really who needs sunscreen inside their bodies? No one!

So in short my advice on sunscreen is the following:

- Before putting on sunscreen, cover up with clothes and hats to protect yourself from harmful UV rays;
- Hang out in the shade rather than direct sun and aim for early morning or late afternoon;
- Wear sunglasses to protect the eyes as well from the harmful UVA and UVB rays. You will protect yourself from possible cataracts as well as from squinting which can cause wrinkles around the eyes later!
- If you must use sunscreen, choose one which is "clean"; this means a rating of less than 5 on the Skin Deep Database and using zinc oxide;
- Use a sunscreen on the face if you will be exposed for longer than 20 minutes in direct sunlight for an extended period of time;
- You may also want to put sunscreen on the hands and decollete (neck and chest area);
- Use a body sunscreen if planning on being at the beach for a long period of time;
- Avoid alcoholic beverages that dehydrate skin and promote burning when outside, and instead sip on antioxidant-rich, iced green tea;
- Put sunscreen on first, then moisturizer, and
- Check the UV Index where you are to know how strong it is.

Harmful sunscreen ingredients

Many ingredients used in sunscreen products are xenoestrogenic meaning that they will interfere with natural hormones. This interference can mean a number of different things from infertility and low sperm count to reproductive diseases and breast cancer in females.

In a study of popular sunscreen ingredients, including benzophenone-3 (Bp-3), homosalate (HMS), 4-methyl-benzylidene camphor (4-MBC), octyl-methoxycinnamate (OMC), and octyl-dimethyl-PABA (OD-PABA), animals exposed to these ingredients experienced an increased proliferation of MCF-7 breast cancer cells. Use of 4-MBC, OMC, and Bp-3 also resulted in an increase in the weight of the uterus, showing that these chemicals affect other reproductive organs, as well. Only one chemical, butyl-methoxydibenzoylmethane (B-MDM), did not result in estrogenic activity.

The following is a partial list of harmful ingredients to avoid when purchasing sunscreen products:

- Avobenzone: Carcinogenic and frequently listed chemical ingredient which only works on UVA rays, not UVB. It breaks down into unknown chemicals when exposed to sunlight and 50-90% of the sunscreen protection is lost after an hour. Once absorbed into the skin it becomes destructive.
- Aminobenzoic acid: Carcinogen implicated in cardiovascular disease.
- Cinoxate: Evidence of skin toxicity.
- Dioxybenzone: Strong evidence of skin toxicity and carcinogen; hormone disruptor and has been found

in waterways, soil and air. Has been shown to have a "gender bender" effect in animals.

- Diazolidinyl urea: Carcinogen, endocrine, central nervous system and brain effects, skin toxicity and compromises the immune system.
- Ecamsule: Carcinogenic.
- Glycols: Often used as moisturizers but once absorbed into the skin, overexposure can cause kidney and liver damage, as well as negative effects on the reproductive system.
- Homosalate: Endocrine disruption.
- Methylparaben: Interferes with genes.
- Octyl salicylate: Broad systemic effects in animals at moderate doses.
- Octocrylene: An active ingredient in most sunscreens it is bioaccumulative, carcinogenic and may cause liver damage.
- Oxybenzone: Carcinogenic and used to aid other chemicals penetrate the skin. It triggers allergic reactions and is considered carcinogenic, a hormone disruptor as well as forms free radicals which cause premature aging. The EWG strongly recommends not using this in anything especially children and yet it is often found in baby sunscreens.
- Octyl Methoxycinnamate (OMC): Is considered phototoxic and is a main chemical used to filter UVB rays. Accumulates in the body, disrupts liver and is a carcinogen.
- Padimate O: Carcinogen.
- Parabens: Including Methyl and Propyl, are used as preservatives in many sunscreens. It acts like oestrogen and increases the number of oestrogen-

sensitive breast cancer cells. Can also disrupt hormonal balance and cause skin rashes, redness, and pain or irritation of the eyes, nose and throat.

- Phenylbenzimidazole: Carcinogen.
- Propylene Glycol: Derived from petroleum, it is highly toxic and can cause eye, nose and throat irritation, neurological and blood disorders.
- Phenoxyethanol: Irritant, carcinogen, and endocrine disruption.
- Retinal Palmitate: A form of vitamin A which creates free radicals when exposed to sunlight. Can become carcinogenic upon sun exposure and may speed up the development of skin tumours and lesions on sun-exposed skin. Vitamin A can cause excess skin growth and cancerous tumours when exposed to sunlight.
- Stearyl and Cetyl Alcohol: Alcohol dries the skin, promotes brown spots and premature skin aging. Can irritate skin, eyes and lungs.
- Sulisobenzone: Strong evidence of skin toxicity, effects sense organs in animals.
- Titanium dioxide: Carcinogen when in nanomaterial form.
- Triethanolamine: Can lead to cancer causing compounds if the sunscreen contains nitrites.
- Zinc Oxide: Bioaccumulative in wildlife, evidence of reproductive toxicity.

This is a scary list!! And as you can see we are exposing ourselves to toxicity with every application of sunscreen! The chemicals interfere with our body's normal systems related to things like our immune and hormone systems. I don't know about you, but I don't want to interfere with that!

Many of these ingredients have not been tested or approved for safety, and that is a scary thought as well! And there has been very little testing as to the bio-accumulative and conjunction with other chemicals. The more chemicals in a sunscreen the great health risk. Many of the kids brands of sunscreen have the same if not MORE harmful ingredients, a disturbing, unethical practice if you ask me.

All of this toxicity is ending up in our bodies and in our environments. And there is little evidence to support that sunscreen is protecting against melanomas. There is research though supporting that these ingredients are carcinogenic. And just so we are clear, carcinogenic means it has been linked directly to causing cancer. So you can see the irony!? Sunscreen is actually causing cancer!

Even though we are using more and more sunscreen every year, skin cancer rates continue to go up. There is little proof that sunscreen helps prevent skin cancer though it may protect from burning and block the harmful UVA and UVB rays. If people focused on taking in enough Vitamin D every day naturally (from the sun for 20 minutes daily), they would do a better job of protecting themselves against cancer. When we cover ourselves up with sunscreen we prevent the beneficial absorption from the sun of Vitamin D which is essential to building up our immune system and therefore protecting against cancer.

So to be clear, I am not against sunscreen, but you have to use the right one and at the right time!

For the acneic teen, be careful with what, when and how they are using the sunscreen and take vitamin D!

Products

We love the Suntegrity Face Sunscreen from California. It has a 1 rating on the Skin Deep Database; it is a professional brand and available on our online store www.myskinsalon.com and other fine spas!

Food sources for sun protection

Believe it or not, there are foods that can help protect us from the sun! Many fruits and vegetables offer sources of vitamins C and E which are proven to protect from the sun's harmful rays.

Other good sources include:

- Beta-carotene: used for years to repair sun-damaged skin; carotenoids are fat-soluble pigments that give oranges and yellows to fruits and flowers. Also found to prevent DNA mutations triggered by the sun. We cannot synthesize carotenoids so we need them from food. Beta carotene converts into vitamin A, essential for skin protection from the sun. Great food sources include carrots, red peppers and mangoes. Excellent vitamin A food sources include paprika, alfalfa, animal livers and fish oils.
- Lutein: found in dark green leafy vegetables and can protect the skin from sun damage
- Green tea polyphenol epigallocatechin-3-gallate (EGCG): these have the ability to prevent sun-induced aging, melanoma and non-melanoma skin cancers.
- Selenium: deficiency in selenium has been linked to sun damage. Food sources include onions, garlic, brazil nuts, chia seeds and other nuts/seeds such as flax.

- Omega 3 fat eicosapentaenoic acid (EPA): reduces skin inflammation caused by UV rays and protects the skin at a cellular level.

It is critical to understand there is a balancing act with sun exposure. You need enough naturally to get your body's requirements for vitamin D, but not too much that you are exposing yourself to the risks of burning, aging or worse, cancer. Read your labels and develop healthy habits in the sun. Be smart and enjoy the sun with care!

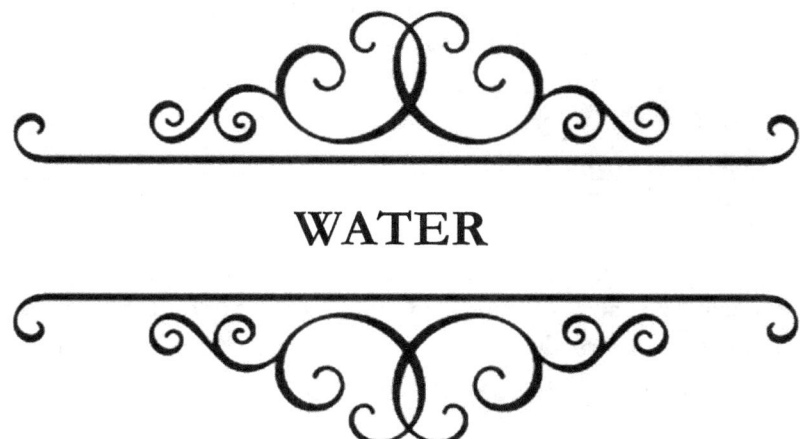

WATER

Water is vitally important to optimal health. It aids with:

- Repair and renewal of cells;
- Removal of waste, toxins and dead skin cells;
- Hydration, in particular the epidermis which must be fed water from underneath, from the dermis;
- Transports oxygen and nutrients to the muscles
- Protects every organ.

For acne sufferers it helps especially with flushing those excess skin cells and for everyone, it helps tone the skin, and leaves it looking dewy, clear and youthful!

Water pollution

One thing we all need to be aware of is that our water is contaminated. It doesn't matter where you live, it has stuff in it that ideally should not be there. A prime example of this is a common and widely used pesticide, pollutant and endocrine-disruptor called Atrazine More than 60 million pounds of it are sprayed on US crops every year, second only to Glyphosate, the active ingredient in Monsanto's troublesome "Roundup". America's own Environmental Protection Agency (EPA) has confirmed that it likely poses a risk to many animal species. An example, low levels of exposure can turn male frogs into females (that produce viable eggs!). Atrazine is commonly found in drinking water as it is actively used on corn crops and thus ends up in our water table. It is linked to breast tumours, delayed puberty and prostate inflammation in animals with some research showing prostate cancer in men.

The bottom line is that you cannot trust your water source and I am advising you to invest in water filtering when you can (more to come on this later). Bad water will lead to toxic overload and therefore inflammation and make acne worse.

How much water to drink

There are several methods used to determine how much water one should drink but the easiest to remember is to not get thirsty! Or use this formula: take your weight and divide by half; this is how many ounces you need to drink daily. As an example, if you weigh 170 pounds, you will need to drink 85 ounces of water a day (or just over 8 cups).

It is better to sip water and not guzzle it; if you guzzle you will be filling your body up and running to the washroom a lot.

There are little tricks your teen can use to get even more hydrated. One is to incorporate Chia seeds into the diet. First, add dry Chia to water until it become gelatinous then add it to a favourite smoothie. Use it as a face mask to soothe inflamed skin too! Try this: add Chia mix to jojoba, honey, lavender and teatree oils, place on skin for 10 minutes.

Please also note that drinking things like juice, sodas or Gatorade doesn't mean your teen is necessarily hydrating his body. Many contain way too much sugar and sodium for starters and can spike insulin (we know now this is very bad for acne).

Caffeine is another issue. Nothing substitutes for water; not juice, alcohol, coffee, tea, etc. The body needs water to perform its functions. The body has water in it right now doing its thing but it will need "new" water in order to do more things such as filtering and bringing out toxins, hydrating cells e.g. brain cells so they function at their best.

Dehydration symptoms

I believe most people are chronically dehydrated. A book by Dr. Batmanghelid called "Water Cures and Drugs Kill" outlines why dehydration is the cause of pain and disease and that the pharmaceutical industry has hidden this information so people will continue to use their drugs. He also mentions that prescription drugs kill more than 250,000 people a year in the US due to faulty prescriptions or just plain use of these drugs. This makes it the third highest killer of people after heart disease and cancer.

Signs of dehydration can include feeling tired, quick to anger, depression, allergies, asthma, and shortness of breath. Our skin can really show dehydration through obvious creases, crow's feet, and the dreaded turkey neck.

Don't wait to get thirsty in order to drink. Just make it part of your teen's daily regimen to sip on water throughout the day using the calculation noted above. One way to know if your teen is drinking enough is to have them look at the colour of their urine. If one is properly hydrated it should be a very pale yellow or almost colourless colour. If it becomes too yellow your teen is dehydrated.

What kind of water to drink

I highly recommend that you invest in a water purifying system of some kind for your home. I am fortunate that where I live we have an abundance of water. Though it comes from nature it is also heavily chlorinated and I just do not want that in my body. Chlorine is a known carcinogenic and so it is important to get impurities like chlorine out of your water.

I do not believe in buying bottled water for two reasons. One we don't know what we are buying and two, we are contributing to pollution through the use of plastic bottles. I recommend the Nikken Mag Water system and you can also invest in a Kangan, though it is very pricy. There are others but my experience has mostly been with Nikken. I also use their shower head filter as we are exposed to so much chlorine through the shower water. As skin is our largest organ, it is absorbed right into our bodies. This is especially important for anyone with skin issues such as acne, eczema, dermatitis or rosacea.

I like to add lemon to my water first thing when I get up as my liver will be happier! I also like to fill up two bottles with my allotted water for the day and keep it nearby so I know where I am am with what I need to drink on a daily basis. It will serve as a great reminder to keep on sipping!

These days I am also a fan of coconut water to replace things like caffeine and sports drinks. Have your teen switch so s/he will get the electrolytes needed. Coconut is known to hydrate quickly so it is ideal if you are in a warm climate and suddenly feel dehydrated.

DAILY HABITS

I t is the small things we do every day that can add up to big changes in areas we would like to change so I put together a list of reminders that may serve your teen well on a daily basis!

Don't pick your face!

It is hard but your teen must not do it! Instead try rubbing ice on pustules or pimples for 5 minutes, twice a day. If your teen can do this when they are first forming they will most likely go away. Your teen can also use Benzoyl Peroxide for this but the surrounding tissue may get very dry. Another idea is to spot treat it with a Q-tip and essential oils such as lavender and teatree. Picking will lead to scars so help them understand the importance of stopping!

Too much drying

People think when they have acne they have to dry their skin out with things like over scrubbing/drying, alcohol or the

sun. This is not the answer and will often result in exacerbating the acne. With active acne, the skin needs to be calmed, cooled and hydrated. Try spritzing in the summer to help cool the skin.

Stop touching the face with the hands!

Another one! Your teen's hands can often be full of dirt, bacteria, oil and other menacing things. When they touch their face with their hands they are spreading it all over their poor face!

Breathe

Breathe work is essential to keeping a body working well and energized. When we get stressed we tend to hold our breath, breathe in a shallow fashion or tighten our chests; this is tough on the body and causes it to tense up. Relax and let everything flow. Your teen's face will look more relaxed and they will feel better which benefits their entire body especially their stress responses (which as we now know can cause acne).

Exercise

We all know exercise is important for a lot of reasons. One of the main is that it moves our lymphatic fluid around the body. Lymph fluid contains toxins so it needs to get out of the body or stagnation happens which results in things like acne, cellulite and other problems such as sinus issues.

Do Yoga

We can all benefit from the practice of yoga. It allows for movement, better balance and focus. It also allows us to set an intention and therefore calms the mind. There are many types of yoga including Vinyasa, Hatha (my favourite), Ashtanga,

Bhakti Flow, Iyenger, Yin and Restorative. Each will offer a different advantage and there are times our bodies need different things. The mind body connection to holistic health is crucial and yoga really helps with this.

Set Intentions

Setting a daily intention will allow for energy to follow thoughts. By focusing on the kind of day your teen would like (hopefully an amazing one!) they can align their being. I like to use the "I am's" which is something Dr Wayne Dyer really spoke of often. I start and end most days with this practice. It reminds me of what I am (and not what I am NOT!). For instance "I am health, I am wealth, I am complete, I am whole". This is great for our bodies and souls!

Show Gratitude

Starting and or ending each day with gratitude will leave your teen feeling better. It is hard to be angry or sad when you are thinking of all the wonderful things in your life to be thankful for. Help your teen develop a ritual s/he can use daily to do this. For me, I end my day, just before I am ready to go to sleep, and I say my thank you's in relation to some of the things that may have happened that day as well as a series of thank you's for the things in my life I love such as the people around me, my family, friends, the work I do, etc. Try it! Your teen will feel better and start to notice subtle changes in how s/he feels!

Hang out with Positive and Like-minded People

Be mindful of the people your teen is spending time with and really start to pay attention to how s/he is and feels around them. Ask them to pay attention when they spent time with someone, to notice how they feel after leaving that person. Do they feel better, worse or the same? If they felt worse and this is a constant thing, you may want to encourage them to minimize exposure to that person. In my life I have stopped friendships because I saw this pattern of feeling down after spending time with certain people, so I stopped spending time with them! Your time is precious and ideally your teen needs to be around people who inspire and energize them so help them be selective!

Also, look to build an alliance of practitioners who can serve your teen in their wellbeing journey. Check them out online, and through referrals and reviews. You want to spend your hard earned money with people who are aligned to you and your teen's wellbeing journey. This can include an Aesthetician, energy healers, massage therapists and more.

Be Open

Life will present your teen with twists and turns on their journey. Encourage them to be open to these experiences and know that they are presenting your teen with an opportunity to grow and learn. Life is not a smooth ride, it will be full of ups and downs, more like a rollercoaster. So, help them to be open to this and love that they get to experience it fully and open!

Look for more than one solution

When problems arrive in life, and we know they will, let your teen know that there will be more than one way to solve them. There is no such thing as failure, just experience. Failures will provide valuable learning experiences and allow your teen to try more than one way to deal with life's issues.

Laughter

Laughter in our lives is so important. It is healing, joyous and produces an energy shift that leaves us feeling better. Encourage your teen to make a point of spending their day doing things that bring them joy, whether it be with friends or work, and take every chance they can to laugh out loud!

A FEW OTHER THINGS TO CONSIDER

Time

Acne sufferers need to give themselves the time it needs to heal their bodies. For some this may mean a month, for others up to 6 months or more. If your teen makes the recommended dietary changes along with a good home care and a few professional sessions to deal with extractions and exfoliation, they should start to see an improvement after 4-6 weeks. If your teen can continue with the program for a full 3 months, s/he will definitely see the changes. It takes patience and courage, but your teen will get there if they do the work and are committed.

Acne Scars

If acne is left untreated it will very likely lead to scarring. This is preventable but your teen must take action as soon as they see their skin changing for the worse. This is why collagen intake is also helpful as it will help to rebuild weak tissue so scarring is minimized or even repaired.

Acne scars can negatively affect a person's confidence. Luckily there are many things that can be done to help. Here are a few helpful hints:

- Seek professional advice as to what can be done about scars; best options are either a Dermatologist or an experienced Aesthetician. Many Aestheticians will offer complimentary consults which will give your teen an idea as to what may be done.

- There are many procedures that can help to reduce scars and promote skin renewal including peels, light therapy and lasers.

- Look to your teen's overall lifestyle and look to ways s/he can improve their overall approach to living in a more healthful way. They will feel better and their confidence will also improve.

- Have them look inside their true being and acknowledge their uniqueness, potential and value of who they are. Your teen needs to work on himself from the inside out to get a healthier self-image. This is where their mindset and self-talk become really important.

- Encourage your teen to respect himself and he will find himself happier and with a better attitude.

- Help your teen change their perspective about the scars, and do not give it attention.

- If their feelings persist do not be afraid to seek professional help in the form of therapy, counselling, etc. Perhaps a session with a

Hypnotherapist may help. Your teen's deep seated issues around beliefs may also be getting in the way and a Hypnotherapist can help with this.

- Look for a support group or Meetup to join like-minded people. Your teen is not alone! There are an estimated 20 million people in the USA who have acne scars! Sharing her experience and toxic emotions can help your teen feel better, more hopeful and peaceful.

Acne scars can have lasting emotional, physical and psychological effects. Encourage your teen to do something about it if it continues to bother them.

The best way to avoid acne scars to begin with is to avoid the behaviour that causes them. Ensure your teen seeks help when their acne worsens e.g. from a grade 1 to 2. Do not think that they can handle what is happening. It is best to ensure they are doing all they can to manage their acne. And secondly, encourage them to stop picking their face!

If they are able to follow these two suggestions your teen will do a lot to avoid acne scarring.

Antibiotics

Many clients who come to see us at our skincare clinic have been to see a dermatologist who generally prescribed antibiotics as the first course of action. Sometimes it works, often it does not. If it did not work the first time, have your teen ask, why keep doing it?

Acne is not a bacteria problem, it is an inherited tendency of too many dead skin cells within the pores. Antibiotics do nothing to address this issue.

If your teen does not need to take antibiotics, don't. Here are more reasons not to take antibiotics:

- A lot of bacteria is becoming drug-resistant;
- MRSA, a superbug, is a very dangerous type of staph infection. It is also very drug resistant to most antibiotics. It is believed to have gotten to this point as a result of the overuse of antibiotics, including the use of antibiotics to treat acne.
- Acne bacteria is now becoming drug-resistant as well. Though it will not kill you, it will become harder to control to achieve clear skin;
- People who use antibiotics are more prone to catch colds, according to a study in the September 2005 issue of Archives of Dermatology. Antibiotics destroy both bad and good bacteria in the gut. This can reduce the body's ability to fight off foreign invaders including bacteria and viruses, hence the increased vulnerability to getting sick more often;.
- In a study published in the Journal of the American Medical Association, heavy antibiotic use may increase a woman's risk of developing breast cancer. The study of 10,000 women over 8 years found that those on the highest amount of antibiotics over the longest period of time were twice as likely to develop breast cancer than those who did not.
- Possible side effects of taking antibiotics includes recurring nausea and heartburn, interference with the useful bacteria in the digestive system, frequent vaginal yeast infections, and possible permanent staining of the teeth.

In relation to other medications, it is important to know that there may be side effects such as depression, low self esteem and even suicide. Make sure your teen has someone they can talk to if they seem to be feeling any of these.

Ultimately we feel the best treatment option for acne is professional consultations to review your teen's current skin state, skincare routine and product use at home, along with professional treatments including regular exfoliation, extraction, assessment, blue LED light, oxygen and coaching. For more severe acne, a doctor's input becomes important.

Your teen's at home regimen could include the topical use of an alpha or beta hydroxy acid which is strong enough to exfoliate but does not burn or irritate the skin, along with an anti-bacterial product that delivers oxygen to the pores. This part is very subjective and requires testing as conditions vary. Patience is also critical as some people will see quicker results than others. Maintaining a positive outlook is also critical.

Accutane

As practitioners in the skincare industry we get very concerned about the use of Accutane (isotretinoin), especially those on repeated use of this dangerous drug (our opinion). While some people do receive a benefit of its use in terms of clear skin, we have to ask ourselves, at what price? Even those who do benefit, their acne usually returns after they stop taking it.

The US Food and Drug Administration (FDA) posted an alert about Accutane in 2005 suggesting that users should closely monitor for serious symptoms and should stop taking Accutane if any appear. These symptoms included:

- Depression;
- Suicidal tendencies;
- Sadness;
- Short tempers and anger;
- Loss of social interaction;
- Psychosis;
- Loss of motivation;
- Changes in appetite;
- Crohn's disease;
- Central nervous system issues;
- Skeletal damage;
- Liver damage;
- Cardiovascular injuries;
- Bone and muscle loss;
- Ulcerative colitis;
- Pancreatitis, and
- Immune system disorders.

In 2002, the FDA Director told a congressional committee that they received over 3,000 reports of adverse psychiatric symptoms along with 170 reports of attempted suicide. Additional risks include birth defects, miscarriage, and fetal death. Women of childbearing age face restricted use of the drug and must be cleared by their physician that they are not pregnant and on at least two forms of birth control.

Roche Holding AG pulled Accutane from the US market after juries awarded at least $33 million in damages to users who blamed the drug for bowel disease. Many are now on colostomy bags for the rest of their lives.

Are these risks really worth it?

CLOSING COMMENTS

My objective with this book was to help young people with acne and their journey through teenagehood into young adulthood. I have a young teenager myself and I want to help him get through this often difficult time with as little pain around his possible acne as possible. I believe acne can hurt young people and their self esteem which has long term effects as they reach adulthood.

Many of the habits I have outlined will serve your teen well as they become an adult. I always tell people that our skin is a reflection of what is going on in our bodies. The habits I have outlined around food, water, stress, sleep and others will help everyone and especially set your teen up for a life of wellbeing and health.

This book has been a journey of discovery for me and a confirmation that the work we do in our clinic can truly help people improve their health and feelings about themselves. My advice to everyone is to be proactive and take an active interest in your health. Do not take everything at face value and look to follow your intuition around what you are doing to and feeding your body.

I welcome any feedback you have on this book. If it has helped you in some way, please let me know! If you have ideas as to how to improve it, let me know that too. I truly am interested in hearing from you! You can contact me in several ways including our web site www.dermabrightclinic.com and the following Social Media platforms:

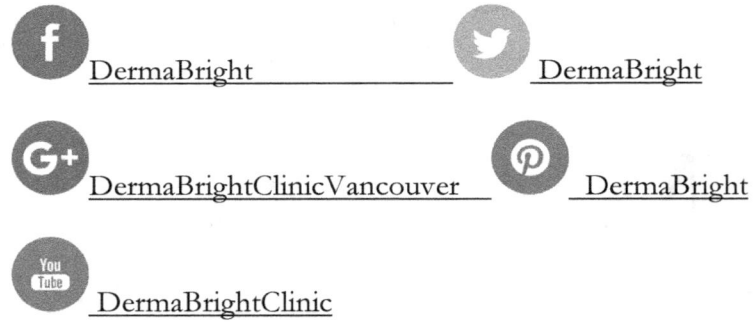

DermaBright   DermaBright

DermaBrightClinicVancouver   DermaBright

DermaBrightClinic

I wish you all well in your journey to better skin, greater health and wellbeing!

Love and Light,

Estrellita Gonzalez

Owner, Derma Bright Clinic and MySkinSalon.com

Owner, She Power Publishing

Queen of Living Clean

RESOURCES

I have put together a few resources here which will help your teen with his or her acne healing journey:

- Vegetable Chart: a reminder of the vegetables we need to be eating;
- Nutritarian Food Plate
- Acne Checklist
- Face Drawing: use this to note the initial state of your teen's face and then use a clean copy once a month to see for yourself the changes and improvements your skin will go through.

Vegetable Chart

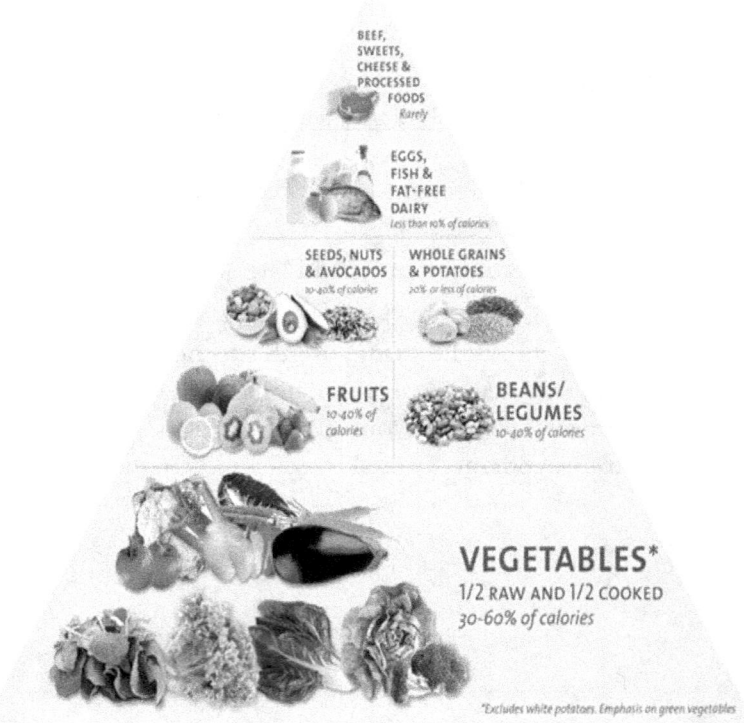

Copyright © 2010 Joel Fuhrman M.D.

Nutritarian Food Plate

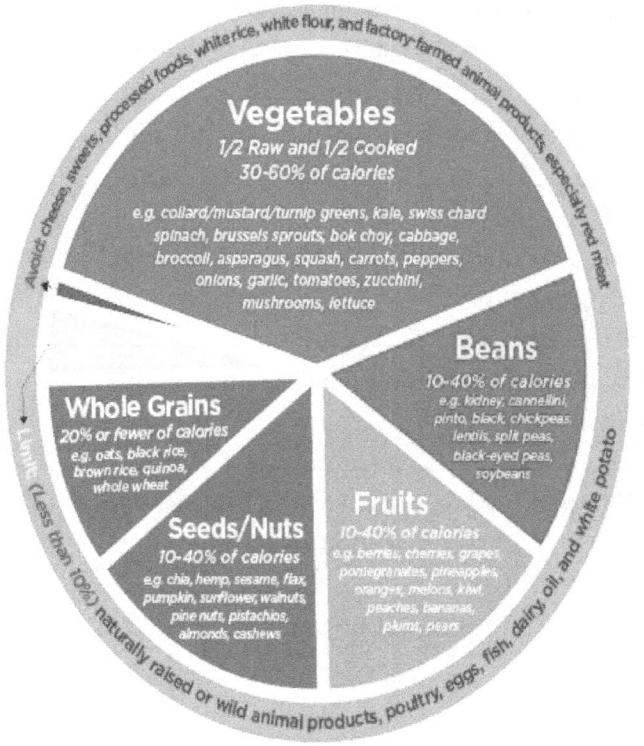

Copyright ©2012 Joel Fuhrman M.D.

Acne Checklist

1	Eat the right foods - vegetables/fruits, protein, & limit processed foods; eat organic where possible
2	Test yourself for food sensitivities and allergies
3	Take supplements - anti-oxidants, esp Vit A & C, , Zinc, fish oils, Probiotics, GLA oils [borage], collagen support
4	Drink adequate clean filtered water - 6-8 glasses a day
5	Detoxify: Juicing, sauna treatments, massage, rebounder, lymphatic treatments
6	Exercise: to get blood flowing and to help move toxins out
7	Invest in a chemical-free, non pore plugging sunscreen and use on your face daily
8	Take Vitamin D supplements or better get from the sun on the rest of your body for 15-20 minutes

9	Use "clean" products - look out for synthetics, chemicals, preservatives, dyes/colours, fragrances
10	Make sure you are using the right products for your skin type and age; get a skin assessment
11	Stick with a skin care routine and use it every day, without fail
12	Exfoliate: daily or at least twice a week - at home - perhaps Microdermabrasion once a month
13	Take time for self-care - small luxuries, meditation, delegation, get a life coach
14	Wash your face twice a day and be gentle on your skin - no scrubbing!
15	Try not to sleep on your tummy or side
16	Don't pick your face - will harm collagen and leave scars!!
17	Test yourself for heavy metals - mercury and lead can lead to skin issues
18	Breathe - make an effort to breathe deeply into your stomach; try Yoga

19	Deal with your stress - talk it out, exercise, meditate, yoga, get a massage
20	Don't smoke EVER
21	Watch your alcohol intake; try and stick to just red wine which has benefits in moderation
22	Sleep - aim for at least 7-8 hours a day (8-10 if a teen); your body repairs itself at night
23	Test your hormones especially if you are mid 40 or up dealing with Acne
24	Get regular facials and peels; your texture will improve and help keep pores small
25	Deal with brown spots, rosacea, scars, etc. before they get worse
26	Use a day and night moisturizer - 2 different ones
27	Take time for proper daily bowel elimination
28	Clean your makeup implements on a regular basis - i.e. brushes etc..
29	Go off all refined sugars, anything white & all Dairy

30	Use warm water for your showers rather than hot; too hot removes beneficial sebum oil
31	Do not use fabric softeners
32	Minimize eating hot & spicy foods
33	Clean your cellphone - it's germs get on your face

Face Drawing

Female

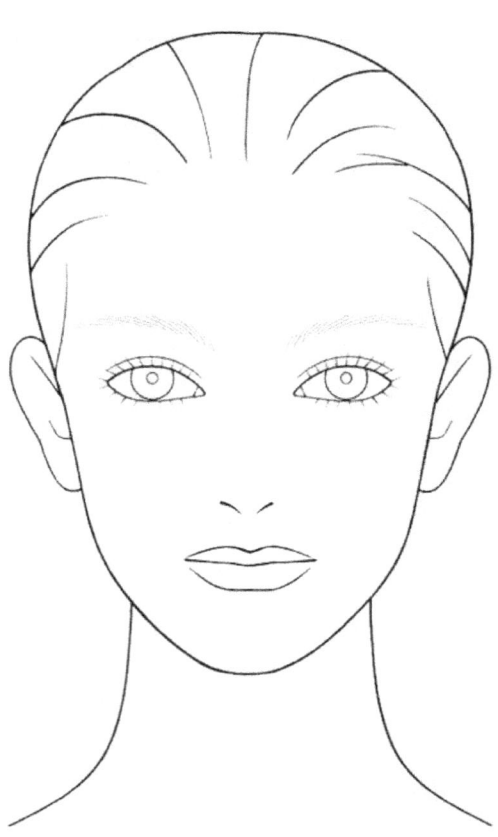

Source: https://www.pinterest.com/KatiaStudio/make-up-by-katia-creative-studiodiy/

Male

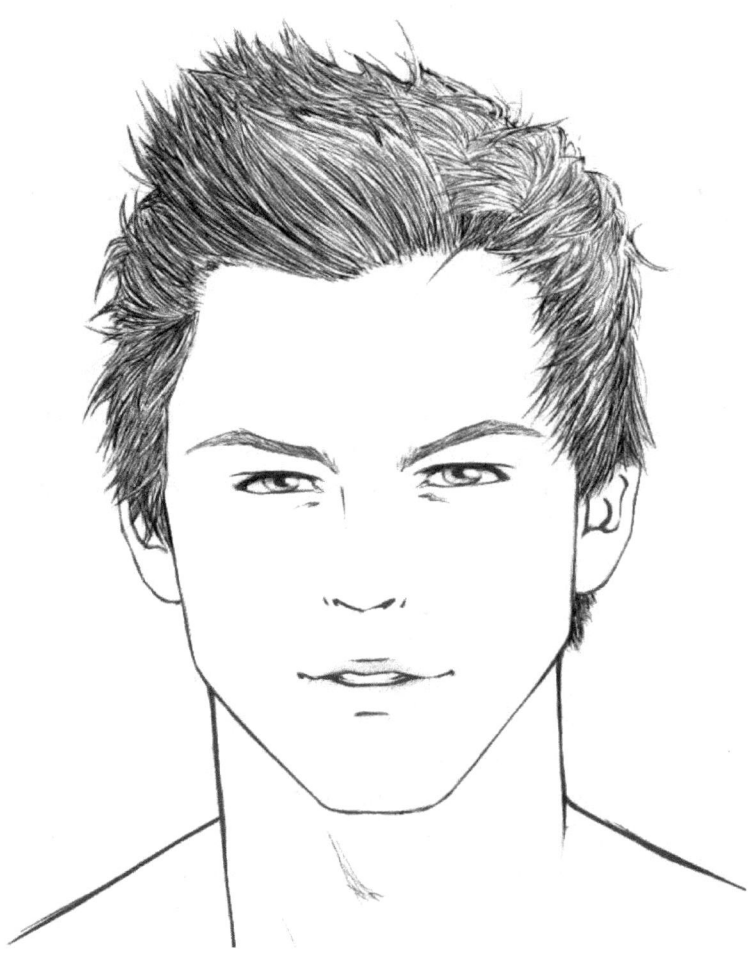

Source: www.sharenoesis.com

SPECIAL OFFERS

As a thank you for reading my book I have a few special offers you are welcome to redeem! Please visit http://dermabrightclinic.com/2016/09/face-your-acne-book-special-offers/ to find out how to get these offers:

- We launched our online store this year - www.myskinsalon.com. Please go to the above link to receive a special coupon code for you to use on our store for clean skincare products and supplements.

- If you are in a rural or remote location it is often difficult to get the professional help you need for your skin so we have a Virtual Assessment available which we do live via Skype or Zoom. Please go to the above link to receive a special coupon code for 25% off this service!

- Could you use a Holistic Nutrition Assessment, virtually? Check out our special offer on the link above or call 604.259.8757, email us on info@dermabrightclinic.com or visit www.dermabrightclinic.com!

- Our DNA can tell us a lot about ourselves. If this is of interest we have a DNA Test. Call 604.259.8757 or email

info@dermabrightclinic.com and mention
"DNA" to receive a $100 off coupon!

REFERENCES

Books & Articles

The Healing Power of Water, Dr Batmanghelidj - Interview by Mike Adams. 2005 Truth Publishing, Ltd.

American Academy of Dermatology: Acne. Costa A, Lage D, Moises TA. **Acne and diet: truth or myth?** *An Bras Dermatol* 2010, **85**:346-353.

Melnik BC, Schmitz G. **Role of insulin, insulin-like growth factor-1, hyperglycaemic food and milk consumption in the pathogenesis of acne vulgaris.** *Exp Dermatol* 2009, **18**:833-841.

Ferdowsian HR, Levin S. **Does diet really affect acne?** *Skin Therapy Lett* 2010, **15**:1-2, 5.

Danby FW. **Diet and acne.** *Clin Dermatol* 2008, **26**:93-96.

Pappas A. **The relationship of diet and acne: A review.** *Dermato Endocrinol* 2009, **1**:262-267.

Logan AC. **Dietary fat, fiber, and acne vulgaris.** *J Am Acad Dermatol* 2007, **57**:1092-1093.

Picardo M, Ottaviani M, Camera E, Mastrofrancesco A. **Sebaceous gland lipids.** *Dermato Endocrinol* 2009, **1**:68-71.

Adebamowo CA, Spiegelman D, Berkey CS, et al. **Milk consumption and acne in adolescent girls.** *Dermatol Online J* 2006, **12**:1.

Adebamowo CA, Spiegelman D, Berkey CS, et al. **Milk consumption and acne in teenaged boys.** *J Am Acad Dermatol* 2008,**58**:787-793.

Adebamowo CA, Spiegelman D, Danby FW, et al. **High school dietary dairy intake and teenage acne.** *J Am Acad Dermatol 2005*, **52**:207-214.

Amer M, Bahgat MR, Tosson Z, et al. **Serum zinc in acne vulgaris.** *Int J Dermatol* 1982, **21**:481-484.

Barclay AW, Petocz P, McMillan-Price J, et al. **Glycemic index, glycemic load, and chronic disease risk--a meta-analysis of observational studies.** *Am J Clin Nutr* 2008, **87**:627-637.

Gnagnarella P, Gandini S, La Vecchia C, Maisonneuve P. **Glycemic index, glycemic load, and cancer risk: a meta-analysis.***Am J Clin Nutr* 2008, **87**:1793-1801.

El-Akawi Z, Abdel-Latif N, Abdul-Razzak K. **Does the plasma level of vitamins A and E affect acne condition?** *Clin Exp Dermatol* 2006, **31**:430-434.

Smith R, Mann N, Makelainen H, et al. **A pilot study to determine the short-term effects of a low glycemic load** diet on hormonal markers of acne: a nonrandomized, parallel, controlled feeding trial. *Mol Nutr Food Res* 2008, **52:**718-726.

Smith RN, Braue A, Varigos GA, Mann NJ. **The effect of a low glycemic load diet on acne vulgaris and the fatty acid composition of skin surface triglycerides.** *J Dermatol Sci* 2008, **50:**41-52.

Smith RN, Mann NJ, Braue A, et al. **A low-glycemic-load diet improves symptoms in acne vulgaris patients: a randomized controlled trial.** *Am J Clin Nutr* 2007, **86:**107-115.

Web links

http://www.google.com/url?q=http%3A%2F%2Fcosmeto logyusa.com%2F7-bad-habits-that-ruin-your-skin%2F HYPERLINK "http://cosmetologyusa.com/7-bad-habits-that-ruin-your-skin/"& HYPERLINK "http://cosmetologyusa.com/7-bad-habits-that-ruin-your-skin/"sa=D HYPERLINK "http://cosmetologyusa.com/7-bad-habits-that-ruin-your-skin/"& HYPERLINK "http://cosmetologyusa.com/7-bad-habits-that-ruin-your-skin/"sntz=1 HYPERLINK "http://cosmetologyusa.com/7-bad-habits-that-ruin-your-skin/"& HYPERLINK "http://cosmetologyusa.com/7-bad-habits-that-ruin-your-skin/"usg=AFQjCNFuZE49-sI1iP1YkjJljGowWxi7qQ '

http://www.skininc.com/treatments/wellness/alternativet herapies/The-Yoga-of-Skin-Care-An-Embodied-Approach-to-Radiance-296762201.html#sthash.2ZAQultq.dpuf

http://www.skininc.com/treatments/wellness/alternativet herapies/The-Yoga-of-Skin-Care-An-Embodied-Approach-to-Radiance-296762201.html

http://www.oprah.com/style/How-to-Get-Great-Skin-Tips-from-Women-with-Beautiful-Skin/4#ixzz2ID0lxZQh

http://www.skininc.com/treatments/wellness/alternativet herapies/The-Yoga-of-Skin-Care-An-Embodied-Approach-to-Radiance-296762201.html#sthash.2ZAQultq.dpuf

http://www.google.com/url?q=http%3A%2F%2Fcosmeto logyusa.com%2F7-bad-habits-that-ruin-your-skin%2F HYPERLINK "http://cosmetologyusa.com/7-bad-habits-that-ruin-your-skin/"& HYPERLINK "http://cosmetologyusa.com/7-bad-habits-that-ruin-your-skin/"sa=D HYPERLINK "http://cosmetologyusa.com/7-bad-habits-that-ruin-your-skin/"& HYPERLINK "http://cosmetologyusa.com/7-bad-habits-that-ruin-your-skin/"sntz=1 HYPERLINK "http://cosmetologyusa.com/7-bad-habits-that-ruin-your-skin/"& HYPERLINK "http://cosmetologyusa.com/7-bad-habits-that-ruin-your-skin/"usg=AFQjCNFuZE49-sI1iP1YkjJljGowWxi7qQ

http://www.oprah.com/style/How-to-Get-Great-Skin-Tips-from-Women-with-Beautiful-Skin/1#ixzz2ID10RCzA

http://www.skininc.com/treatments/wellness/alternativet herapies/The-Yoga-of-Skin-Care-An-Embodied-Approach-to-Radiance-296762201.html

https://mail.google.com/mail/u/0/?shva=1#inbox/139a0 6723e3e2a24

http://www.drfuhrman.com/library/diet_acne.aspx ::

www.truthpublishing.com

www.watercure.com

www.nafhim.org

www.beautytruth.com

others in how to live a cleaner lifestyle in order to lessen the toxic load in our daily lives.

Estrellita lives in Vancouver, BC Canada with her teenage son and enjoys many things including health/wellness, travel, food/wine and reading. Feel free to reach her on her About page: https://about.me/estrellitagonzalez or on Facebook!

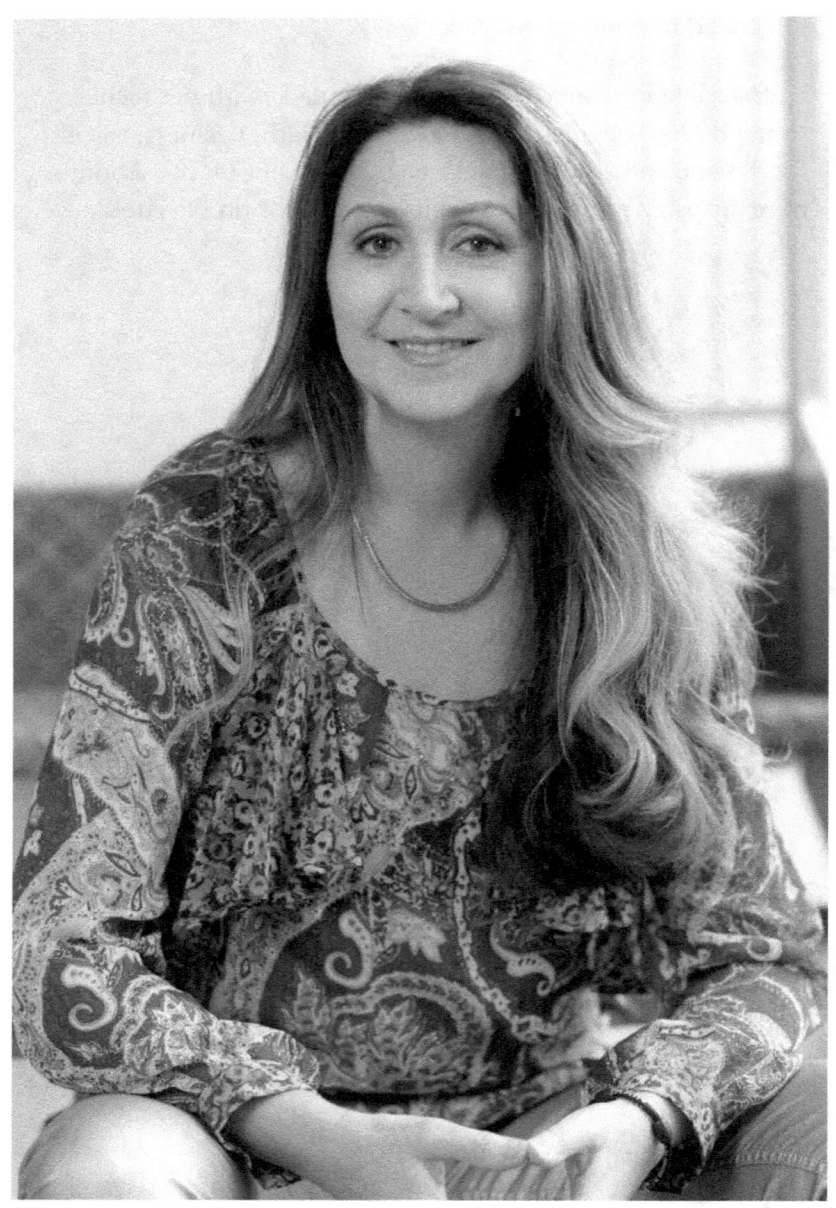